Cystic Fibrosis Reversed

Artour Rakhimov

Dr. Artour Rakhimov

Copyright ©2013-2018 Artour Rakhimov.

All rights reserved.

This book is copyrighted. It is prohibited to copy, lend, adapt, electronically transmit, or transmit by any other means or methods without prior written approval from the author. However, the book may be borrowed by family members.

Disclaimer

The content provided herein is for information purposes only and not intended to diagnose, treat, cure or prevent cystic fibrosis or any other chronic disease. Always consult your doctor or health care provider before making any medical decisions). The information herein is the sole opinion of Dr. Artour Rakhimov and does not constitute medical advice. These statements have not been evaluated by Ontario Ministry of Health. Although every effort has been made to ensure the accuracy of the information herein, Dr. Artour Rakhimov accepts no responsibility or liability and makes no claims, promises, or guarantees about the accuracy, completeness, or adequacy of the information provided herein and expressly disclaims any liability for errors and omissions herein.

Cystic Fibrosis
TABLE OF CONTENTS

PREFACE..5
INTRODUCTION: HYPOXIA, CYSTIC FIBROSIS, AND CHRONIC DISEASES....................6
1. HYPOXIA CONTROLS CYSTIC FIBROSIS TRANSMEMBRANE CONDUCTANCE
REGULATOR (CFTR)..7
2. OXYGEN TRANSPORT IN CYSTIC FIBROSIS..10
   2.1 Minute ventilation in cystic fibrosis patients at rest...............10
   2.2 Breathing frequency in cystic fibrosis.......................................11
3. EFFECTS OF CHRONIC HYPERVENTILATION ON OXYGEN TRANSPORT..................13
   3.1 Hyperventilation with normal lungs..13
   3.2 Hyperventilation causes problems with ventilation-perfusion...............16
   3.3 Additional effects of mouth breathing and hyperventilation on airways and mucus formation in cystic fibrosis................21
   3.4 Nocturnal hypoxemia or nocturnal oxygen desaturation........26
4. CAN AUTOMATIC BREATHING BE RETRAINED?..29
   4.1 Hyperventilation provocation test..30
   4.2 What are the effects of breathing training on people with CF?...........31
   4.3 Clinical trials of the Buteyko breathing technique..................32
5. BODY OXYGEN TEST, BREATHING PATTERNS, MORNING CP........................35
   5.1 How to Measure Body Oxygen Level (DIY Test).......................35
   5.2 Breathing patterns and body oxygenation................................38
   5.3. Morning CP: your main health test...39
6. CLINICAL EXPERIENCE OF RUSSIAN DOCTORS IN RELATION TO CYSTIC FIBROSIS..41
7. BREATHING EXERCISES FOR HIGHER CP..44
   7.1 Buteyko breathing method..44
   7.2 Frolov breathing device..45
   7.3 Amazing DIY breathing device...46
   7.4 Breathing exercises for people with cystic fibrosis..................47
   7.5 Oxygen Remedy online webinars...48
8. LIFESTYLE PROGRAM FOR HIGH BODY OXYGEN IN CF...............................49
   8.1 Morning CP is the main health parameter in cystic fibrosis..................49
   8.2 Sleeping positions..51
   8.3 Methods to prevent back sleeping..52
   8.4 Sleeping in a sitting position: highest body oxygen results.....52
   8.5 Nose breathing 24/7..53
   8.6 Key physical activity factors that improve cell oxygen levels.............56
   8.7 List of common factors for higher morning CP.......................57
   8.8 Diet and meals..58
   8.9 Focal infections..59

8.10 Earthing: Get Grounded to Earth..59
8.11 No acute HV (hyperventilation)...60
8.12 Additional factors..60
8.13 Yoga is useful too (if you know how to breathe)....................61
9. YOUR PROGRAM TO DEFEAT CYSTIC FIBROSIS.....................................63
9.1 Severe and moderate cystic fibrosis..63
9.2 Mild cystic fibrosis..64
9.3 Your ultimate health goal is to have more than 50 s for the body oxygen test 24/7..65
RESOURCES...68
BIBLIOGRAPHY..69
ABOUT THE AUTHOR: DR. ARTOUR RAKHIMOV.....................................79

Preface

In this groundbreaking book on cystic fibrosis, Dr. Artour Rakhimov analyzes dozens of western medical research studies related to causes of cystic fibrosis, effects of low body oxygen content on the human body, breathing parameters in people with cystic fibrosis, oxygen transport in people with cystic fibrosis, and successful clinical experience of Soviet and Russian medical doctors in dealing with cystic fibrosis.

Dr. Artour Rakhimov provides a blueprint and his own fascinating experience related to successful elimination of major symptoms of cystic fibrosis in his students using natural self-oxygenation methods based on breathing normalization or breathing in accordance with medical norms.

This medical program is largely developed by Russian and Soviet Buteyko breathing doctors, and it is based on a simple DIY body oxygen test. The suggested therapies address all those lifestyle factors that influence body oxygenation and suggest breathing exercises that increase body oxygenation.

Dr. Artour Rakhimov

Introduction: hypoxia, cystic fibrosis, and chronic diseases

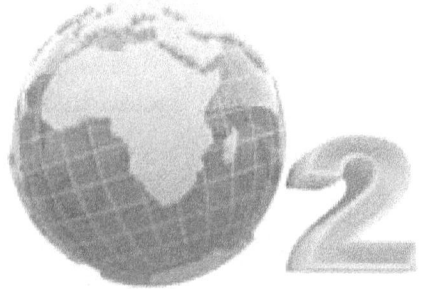

"All chronic pain, suffering and diseases are caused from a lack of oxygen at the cell level."

Professor AC Guyton, MD, Textbook of Medical Physiology*

* World's most widely used medical textbook of any kind
* World's best-selling physiology book

With the advance of any chronic disease, cystic fibrosis included, oxygen content in body and brain cells progressively decreases. Sometimes low cellular oxygen content is the proven driving force of major symptoms and features of diseases (e.g., as in cases of cancer, asthma, bronchitis, and heart disease). For other conditions, tissue hypoxia or low body O2 is an acknowledged accompanying factor. Indeed, for advanced stages of many chronic diseases, cell oxygenation becomes so low that providing pure oxygen is a common mainstream medical treatment to prolong one's life. CF (cystic fibrosis) is no exception.

1. Hypoxia controls cystic fibrosis transmembrane conductance regulator (CFTR)

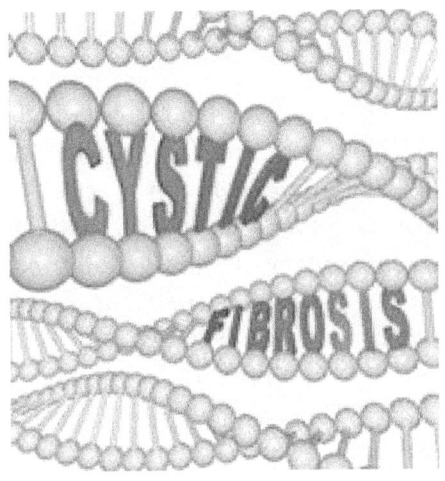

As we learned above, hyperventilation and resultant cell hypoxia are normal in people with CF. Tissue hypoxia leads to overexpression of hypoxia inducible factor-1 (HIF-1), an oxygen-sensitive transcriptional activator, which plays a crucial role in cellular adaptation to reduced oxygen availability. Microbiological studies suggest that HIF-1 (representing oxygen availability) controls the expression of cystic fibrosis transmembrane conductance regulator (CFTR). This conclusion was found in the following articles.

American scientists from the Department of Medicine at the University of Alabama (Birmingham) tested the effects of cell oxygenation on CFTR in vitro. The title of their article in the *American Journal of Physiology and Cell Physiology*, states that *Improved oxygenation promotes CFTR maturation and trafficking in MDCK monolayers* (Bebök et al, 2001). In their abstract, the researchers wrote, "*Together, our data indicate that improved cellular oxygenation can increase endogenous CFTR maturation and/or trafficking*".

Another group of US scientists from Alabama (Department of Genetics, Fleming James Cystic Fibrosis Research Center, University of Alabama at Birmingham) was concerned about the *Role of oxygen availability in CFTR expression and function* (Guimbellot et al, 2008). Their abstract suggests, "... *In the present study, we investigated regulation of CFTR mRNA during oxygen restriction, examined effects of hypoxic signaling on chloride transport across cell monolayers, and related these findings to a possible role in the pathogenesis of chronic hypoxic lung disease. CFTR mRNA, protein, and function were robustly and reversibly altered in human cells in relation to hypoxia. In mice subjected to low oxygen in vivo, CFTR mRNA expression in airways, gastrointestinal tissues, and liver was repressed. CFTR mRNA expression was also diminished in pulmonary tissues taken from hypoxemic subjects at the time of lung transplantation. Environmental factors that induce hypoxic signaling regulate CFTR mRNA and epithelial Cl(-) transport in vitro and in vivo.*"

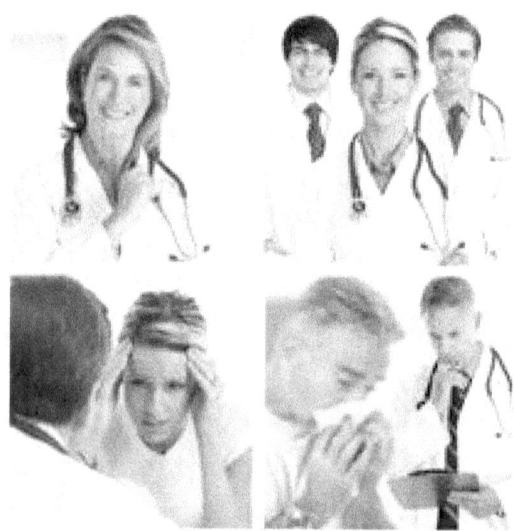

One year later, in 2009, German scientists from the Hanover Medical High School also supported the idea that *Hypoxia inducible factor-1 (HIF-1)-mediated repression of cystic fibrosis transmembrane conductance regulator (CFTR) in the intestinal epithelium* (Zheng et al, 2009). They wrote, " ... *Consequently, HIF-1 overexpressing cells*

exhibited significantly reduced transport capacity in colorimetric Cl(-) efflux studies, altered short circuit measurements, and changes in transepithelial fluid movement. Whole-body hypoxia in wild-type mice resulted in significantly reduced small intestinal fluid and HCO(3)(-) secretory responses to forskolin. Experiments performed in Cftr(-/-) and Nkcc1(-/-) mice underlined the role of altered CFTR expression for these functional changes, and work in conditional HIF-1 mutant mice verified HIF-1-dependent CFTR regulation in vivo. In summary, our study clarifies CFTR regulation and introduces the concept of a HIF-1-orchestrated response designed to regulate ion and fluid movement across hypoxic intestinal epithelia".

Therefore, we can now state that reduced oxygen availability in body cells plays the central role in abnormal work of the CFTR protein that causes formation of salty viscous mucus (due to abnormal transport of chloride and sodium ions and water caused by the CFTR mutation protein). This leads to the development and pathogenesis of CF, where dysfunctional mucus harbors pathogens and promotes respiratory infections and pathological gastrointestinal flora.

Conclusions. Abnormal work of ionic pumps that took place in people with developing cystic fibrosis can take place only due to low oxygen levels in tissues. While all people experience more problems with these tiny pumps to transport sodium, chloride and other ions, people with cystic fibrosis have an additional genetic component that worsens transfer of ions across the epithelial layers in the lungs and GI tract.

In short, if you have reduced body O2 and CFTR gene, you will develop cystic fibrosis since pumping ions requires normal cell oxygenation. If your body O2 stores are normal or high, you will not suffer from effects of the defective cystic fibrosis gene.

Now let us focus on the causes of reduced oxygen levels in people with CF.

Dr. Artour Rakhimov

2. Oxygen Transport in Cystic Fibrosis

Oxygen is delivered to body cells via breathing. Hence, we have to analyze the respiratory parameters and breathing patterns in people with CF. What is wrong with breathing in people with cystic fibrosis?

2.1 Minute ventilation in cystic fibrosis patients at rest

This Table summarizes results of 14 studies performed on healthy subjects and 8 studies related to minute ventilation in cystic fibrosis.

Condition	Minute ventilation	Number of patients	References
Normal breathing	6 L/min	-	Medical textbooks
Healthy subjects	6-7 L/min	>400	Normal Minute Ventilation
Cystic fibrosis	15 L/min	15	Fauroux et a, 2006
Cystic fibrosis*	13 (±2) L/min	10	Bell et al, 1996
Cystic fibrosis	10 L/min	11	Browning et al, 1990
Cystic fibrosis	11-14 L/min	6	Tepper et al, 1983
Cystic fibrosis*	10 L/min	10	Ward et al, 1999
CF and diabetes*	10 L/min	7	Ward et al, 1999
Cystic fibrosis	16 L/min	7	Dodd et al, 2006
Cystic fibrosis	18 L/min	9	McKone et al, 2005

Some studies indicated the abnormal average weight of their subjects. As a result, minute ventilation for 2 studies (Bell et al, 1996) and (Ward et al, 1999) was adjusted to normal weight (70 kg).

Available medical research suggests that a typical person with mild CF breathes at rest from about 10 to 18 liters of air per minute instead of 6 L/min (the medical norm). Therefore, they suffer from chronic hyperventilation (or breathing more than the medical norm). Note that numerous studies have found that modern healthy people have light and easy breathing at rest, with only about 6-7 L/min for their minute ventilation.

2.2 Breathing frequency in cystic fibrosis

Furthermore, many medical professionals have noticed that breathing frequency or respiratory rate is abnormally high in cystic fibrosis. This is reflected in the title of the publication by American doctors from the Department of Medicine of the University of Texas Health Science Center in Houston, Texas in the Chest magazine *Importance of respiratory rate as an indicator of respiratory dysfunction in patients with cystic fibrosis*. The title suggests respiratory frequency in cystic fibrosis correlates with the degree of pathological changes in the lungs. (Note that up to 80% of people with CF die due to respiratory failure.)

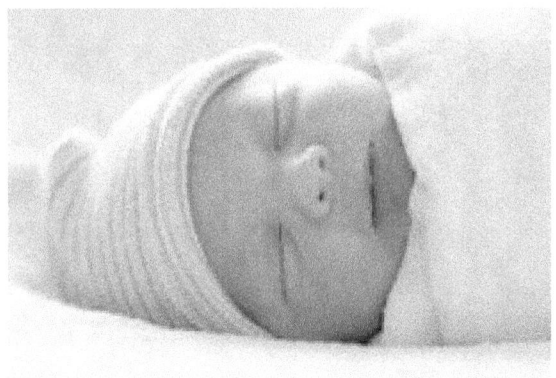

Even infants with CF have higher respiratory frequency in comparison with matched healthy infants. While comparing 95 healthy infants with 47 infants with CF of similar age (39-40 weeks gestational age), sex, ethnicity and proportion exposed to maternal smoking were recruited, it was found that CF infants had a significantly greater respiratory rate (almost 6 more breaths per minute) and elevated minute ventilation as well: 424 ml/kg for infants with CF and 313 ml/kg for healthy infants (Ranganathan et al, 2003).

These measurements suggest that abnormal respiratory parameters, related to chronic hyperventilation with elevated respiratory frequency, appear in people with the CF gene at an early age. Clinical observations also reveal that increased breathing frequency contributes to increased rib cage - abdominal muscular discoordination (upper chest breathing), as is common in CF (see references below).

Chronic hyperventilation found in CF occurs because of increased respiratory frequency and tidal volume. In other words, people with CF breathe faster and deeper than the medical norms. Since metabolic rate and CO_2 production rates are relatively fixed parameters, there is one immediate effect of alveolar hyperventilation in people with CF: alveolar hypocapnia or low levels of CO_2 in the airways and lungs.

3. Effects of chronic hyperventilation on oxygen transport

Let us consider the range of immediate and long-term effects caused by chronic hyperventilation in an otherwise healthy person who has previously had normal breathing parameters.

Chronic hyperventilation (overbreathing) suppresses the oxygen content in cells. There are two different mechanisms of suppression that depend on transport of oxygen in the lungs or ventilation-perfusion ratio.

3.1 Hyperventilation with normal lungs

The most common mechanism of reduced oxygen delivery occurs when there are no problems with the lungs, as in typical cases of heart disease, cancer, diabetes, and light forms of CF. In this case (normal lungs), hyperventilation leads to arterial hypocapnia (reduced CO2), which results in two effects:

A. **Heavy breathing and low CO2 leads to vasoconstriction** or spasm of smooth muscles in arteries and arterioles that causes reduced blood flow or perfusion of all vital organs.

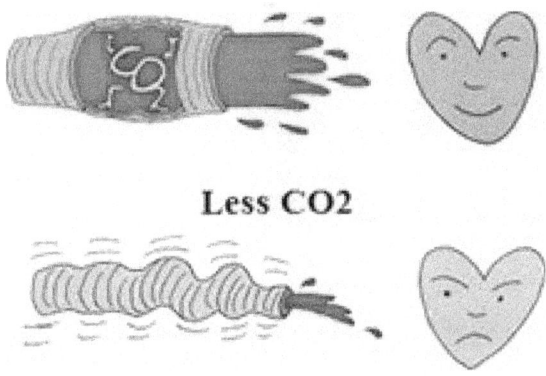

Less CO2

There are numerous studies that proved this effect on:

- brain (Fortune et al, 1995; Karlsson et al, 1994; Liem et al, 1995; Macey et al, 2007; Santiago & Edelman, 1986; Starling & Evans, 1968; Tsuda et al, 1987)

- heart (Coetzee et al, 1984; Foëx et al, 1979; Karlsson et al, 1994; Okazaki et al, 1991; Okazaki et al, 1992; Wexels et al, 1985)

- liver (Dutton et al, 1976; Fujita et al, 1989; Hughes et al, 1979; Okazaki, 1989)

- kidneys (Karlsson et al, 1994; Okazaki, 1989)

- spleen (Karlsson et al, 1994)

- colon (Gilmour et al, 1980).

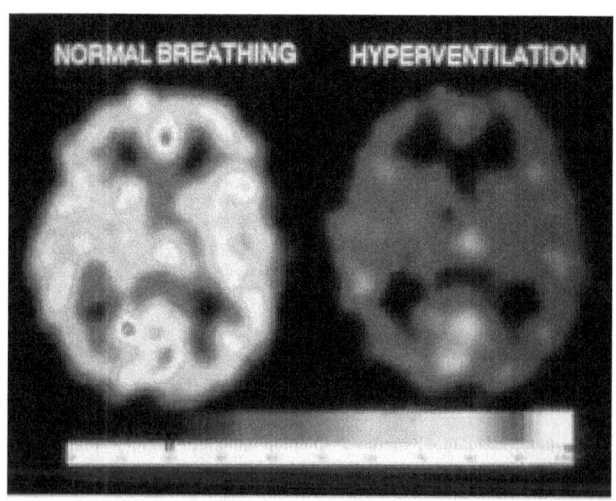

Effects of 1 minute of voluntary hyperventilation on brain oxygen levels (vasoconstriction due to lack of CO2)

Cystic Fibrosis

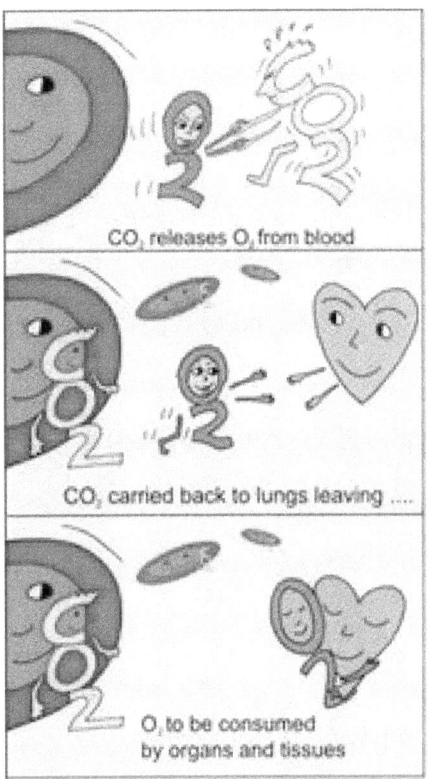

B. The suppressed Bohr effect - low CO2 causes the increased affinity between hemoglobin and oxygen molecules that hampers release of oxygen in tissues (Carter & Grønlund, 1983; diBella et al, 1996; Dzhagarov & Kruk, 1996; Grant, 1982; Jensen, 2004; Kister et al, 1998; Lapennas, 1983; Tyuma, 1984).

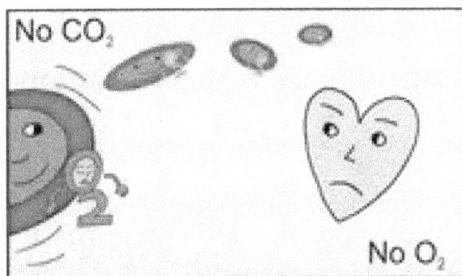

These two effects are independent from each other, but both reduce oxygen transport to cells. As a result, it is a proven fact that hyperventilation reduces cell oxygen level in vital organs of the human body, including:

- brain (Brown, 1953; Kennealy et al, 1980; Liem et al, 1995; Lum, 1975; Lum, 1982; Macey et al, 2007; Litchfield, 2003; Santiago & Edelman, 1986; Skippen et al, 1997; Starling & Evans, 1968; Tsuda et al, 1987)

- heart (Foëx et al, 1979; Karlsson et al, 1994; Okazaki et al, 1991; Okazaki et al, 1992; Wexels et al, 1985)

- liver (Fujita et al, 1989; Hughes et al, 1979; Okazaki, 1989)

- kidneys (Karlsson et al, 1994; Okazaki, 1989)

- spleen (Karlsson et al, 1994)

- colon (Guzman et al, 1999)

- systemic or body tissues in general (Laffey & Kavanagh, 2002; Nunn, 1987).

Note that hyperventilation may not result in hypocapnia (advanced stages of cystic fibrosis, asthma, COPD, etc.) due to ventilation-perfusion mismatch and too high CO_2 in the arterial blood (hypercapnia), but the main driving force for cell hypoxia and destructions of the lungs remains the same: alveolar hyperventilation or too low CO_2 in the lungs.

3.2 Hyperventilation causes problems with ventilation-perfusion

Modern research suggests that alveolar hypocapnia (low CO_2 in the lungs) causes various negative effects on the respiratory system, airways and lungs of normal subjects and people with cystic fibrosis. The adverse effects include:

Cystic Fibrosis

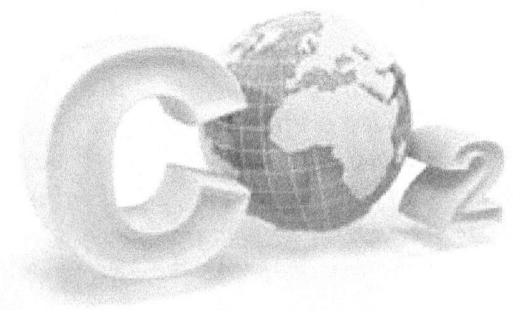

A. Bronchoconstriction, which is a normal physiological reaction to alveolar hyperventilation present in all people (Jamison et al, 1987; O'Cain et al, 1979; Sterling, 1968). However, when hypocapnic bronchoconstriction is combined with chronic tissue hypoxia, the effects are different. Chronic hypoxia leads to anaerobic cellular respiration in mitochondria that causes the production of reactive oxygen species (free radicals) and chronic inflammation.

B. Chronic inflammation, according to medical cystic fibrosis research, is the pivotal point that exacerbates this disease because inflammatory mechanisms in CF airways lead to pulmonary complications which are the most serious complications in cystic fibrosis (e.g., Döring & Worlitzsch, 2000). According to recent biomedical research, chronic inflammation is either associated with or even caused by tissue hypoxia. Medical biologists have finally been able to pinpoint the mechanism. Among the key driving forces of chronic inflammation, according to recent research studies, are pro-inflammatory transcription factors, such as nuclear factor kappa B (NF-kappaB) and activator protein (AP)-1 (Safronova & Morita, 2010; Ryan et al, 2009), and hypoxia-inducible factor 1 (Imtiyaz & Simon, 2010; Sumbayev & Nicholas, 2010). The link between tissue hypoxia and chronic inflammation is so strong, that there are dozens of recent research publications that use the term "hypoxic inflammation".

C. Immunosuppression is a normal result of chronic hypoxia (Sitkovsky, 2009; Hatfield et al, 2009). Here is a part of the recent abstract from one of these studies, "... *Here, we attract attention to the possibility of iatrogenic exacerbation of immune-mediated tissue damage as a result of the unintended weakening of the tissue-protecting, hypoxia-adenosinergic pathway. These immunosuppressive, anti-inflammatory pathways play a critical and nonredundant role in the protection of normal tissues from collateral damage during an inflammatory response. We believe that it is the tissue hypoxia associated with inflammatory damage that leads to local inhibition of overactive immune cells by activating A2AR and A2BR and stabilizing HIF-1alpha. We show in an animal model of acute lung injury that oxygenation (i.e., inspiring supplemental oxygen) reverses tissue hypoxia and exacerbates ongoing inflammatory lung tissue damage...*" (Hatfield et al, 2009).

D. Lung injury, according to Canadian biomedical researchers, is proportional to the degree of alveolar hypocapnia (Laffey et al, 2000; Laffey et al, 2003). Another medical study suggested, according to its title, that *Airway hypocapnia increases microvascular leakage in the guinea pig trachea* (Reynolds et al, 1992) worsening airways injury. While evaluating effects of alveolar hypocapnia on ventilation-perfusion heterogeneity, it was found that "*Hypocapnia worsens arterial blood oxygenation and increases VA/Q heterogeneity in canine pulmonary edema*" (Domino et al, 1993), where VA/Q is the ventilation-perfusion ratio.

What are the possible solutions? "Deliberate elevation of $PaCO_2$ (therapeutic hypercapnia) protects against lung injury induced by lung reperfusion and severe lung stretch" (Laffey et al, 2003). Note that, according to many studies, breathing CO_2-rich air does not improve blood oxygenation and ventilation-perfusion ratio because CO_2 is a powerful respiratory stimulant causing increased minute ventilation that can mechanically worsen existing inflammation and lung injury. In order to be effective, higher alveolar CO_2 content should not be accompanied by excessive mechanical stress.

Cystic Fibrosis

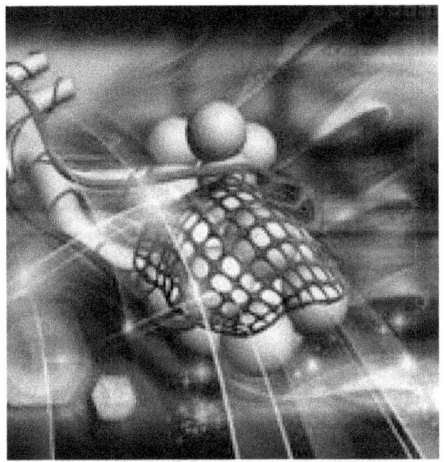

Hence, even when the lungs are not involved, chronic hyperventilation naturally leads to systemic cell hypoxia, bronchoconstriction, chronic inflammation, immunosuppression, frequent respiratory infections and other pathological processes in the lungs that can worsen oxygen transport and increase CO_2 retention.

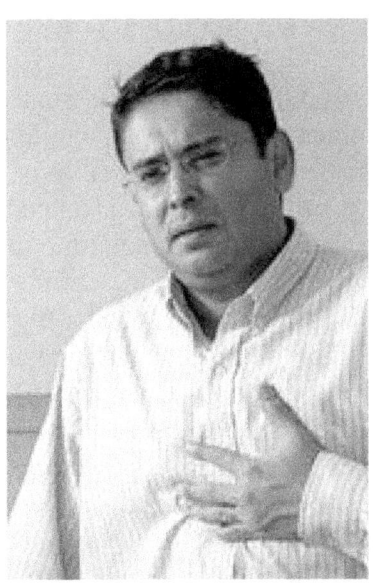

E. Impairment of thoraco-abdominal mechanics (or predominantly upper chest breathing) is a normal result of worsening cell oxygenation, chronic inflammation of airways, and reduced ventilation-perfusion ratio. This effect is common for obstructive lung diseases, while some studies found that contribution of chest breathing correlates with degree of CF (Szeinberg et al, 1985; Pinet et al, 2003; Hart et al, 2004).

Probably, the presence of the faulty CFTR gene makes the situation with diaphragmatic breathing worse, as the title of a recent study suggests *Lack of CFTR in skeletal muscle predisposes to muscle wasting and diaphragm muscle pump failure in cystic fibrosis mice* (Divangahi et al, 2009). The main reason for the diaphragmatic weakness is the hypoxic inflammatory environment for muscle cells of the diaphragm.

These observations suggest that development and maintenance of diaphragmatic breathing 24/7 should be a part of any rehabilitative therapy for any stage of CF, while children with CF must learn simple diaphragmatic breathing techniques (preferably, the Buteyko reduced breathing exercise) as early as possible.

Summary: Effects of chronic hyperventilation on normal lungs

Due to a variety of adverse effects on lung tissue, chronic hyperventilation can result in development of lung pathologies (severe asthma, bronchitis, emphysema, bronchiectasis, bronchiolitis, tuberculosis, and so forth), mild and more advanced forms of CF included. Hampered gas exchange in the lungs (due to airway collapse, modification and destruction of alveoli, chronic inflammation, mucus and liquid in airways and lungs and other abnormalities) leads to lower O_2 and higher CO_2 tensions in the arterial blood (hypoxemia and hypercapnia or CO_2 retention). Worsened ventilation-perfusion ratio immediately causes tissue hypoxia. It is, therefore, common that people with advanced stages of these lung pathologies are candidates for supplemental oxygen. Bear in mind that oxygen therapies work mostly due to the greatly increased amount of oxygen freely dissolved in blood plasma.

Note about breathing pure oxygen. In normal conditions, up to about 98% of all oxygen is combined with red blood cells, while only about 2% of O2 is freely dissolved in plasma. Breathing pure oxygen increases the amount of free oxygen about 5 times, thus, saving the lives of people, but providing mild chronic stress for the lungs due to oxidative stress or the generation of reactive oxygen species (free radicals). Leading respiratory specialists share the same (negative) opinion in relation to pure oxygen therapies and hyperbaric oxygen therapies which may increase oxygenation in under-ventilated portions of the lungs, but are destructive in relation to the functioning parts of the lungs.

3.3 Additional effects of mouth breathing and hyperventilation on airways and mucus formation in cystic fibrosis

Mouth breathing in cystic fibrosis

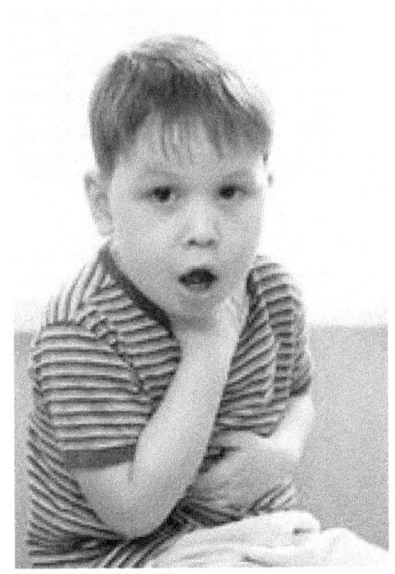

Oral breathing is very common in children and adults with cystic fibrosis (Fernald et al, 1990; Brihaye et al, 1997). The problem appears at a very young age. As it was found by Ramsey & Richardson (1992), " ... *the vast majority of patients with cystic fibrosis develop sinus disease with panopacification of the sinuses present in 90% to 100% of patients older than 8 months of age.*" The common effects of mouth breathing and chronic sinusitis are a loss of the sense of smell, deformities of the external nasal skeleton, and headaches, while up to 20% of patients eventually require surgical treatment of their sinuses (Ramsey & Richardson, 1992).

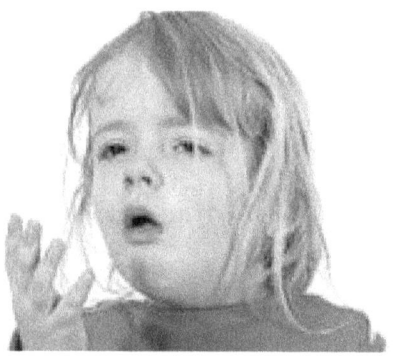

A group of Italian researchers in their article *Orocraniofacial changes in young subjects with cystic fibrosis* suggested that orofacial changes were linked with habitual mouth breathing of young cystic fibrosis people: "...Even if causes can be hardly distinguished from effects, the role of the juvenile oral breathing in these cases seems to be any way undeniable with statistically significant results" (Gola et al, 1989).

A group of Swedish orthodontists in their study *Craniofacial morphology in children with cystic fibrosis* noted that, "... The cystic fibrosis group showed open bite, decreased posterior facial height, increased mandibular and craniocervical inclination" (Hellsing et al, 1992).

Mouth breathing causes drying of airways

What are the effects of habitual hyperventilation through the mouth? A study conducted in the Department of Pediatrics at Case Western Reserve University (Cleveland, Ohio) measured effects of the breathing route on humidity and surface temperature in airways of normal and CF subjects. During nose breathing, the nasal passages are designed to humidify and warm up the incoming flow of air. Mouth breathing leads to drying and cooling of bronchi and bronchioles. For example, during inspiration, the relative humidity at the pharynx for nose breathing was about 95%, while for mouth breathing it was only 75% (Primiano et al, 1988). Hence, mouth breathing requires about 5 times more water from bronchi and bronchioles in order to achieve 100% humidity. (It is unlikely that alveoli significantly contribute to humidification of inhaled air.) These doctors observed that, "... *These data suggest that when the rate of evaporation is sufficiently high, the rate-limiting step may be water transport through the mucosal tissue and/or secretions. At least for the upper airways, this rate limitation is more evident for CF patients than for normal subjects.*"

Hyperventilation and mouth breathing causes overcooling of airways

An additional effect of chronic hyperventilation relates to overcooling of airways, especially in cases of oral breathing. While measuring temperature of airways during pulmonary and hyperventilation tests, a group of Italian doctors discovered that hyperventilation induced a significant temperature loss (Vitacca et al, 1994). The aim of their study was to test the usefulness of hygroscopic condenser humidifiers on secretion and on inspired gas temperature in tracheostomized patients. These Italian doctors found that hygroscopic condenser humidifiers have positive effects of thickness and coloring of mucosal secretions: "*Statistically significant differences were found in thickness and coloring of secretions between the two groups during the period of 10 days. Group 2 showed a significantly greater trend in number of bacteria than Group 1. The group with the hygroscopic condenser humidifier showed respiratory function improvement over time for forced expiratory volume in one second (FEV1) and tidal volume (VT), maximal inspiratory pressure (MIP), and maximal voluntary ventilation (MVV) in comparison to the control group, who did not.*" In conclusion, they write that hygroscopic condenser humidifiers can be useful, among other things, to "*heat inspiratory airflow, possibly protecting against temperature loss during a hyperventilation test*".

These results suggest that hyperventilation in cystic fibrosis also leads to overcooling of airways. It is known that even a slight drop in temperatures of airways can lead to immune dysfunction and possible infections. Overcooling may also contribute to thickness and coloring of sputum, as the above study suggested.

Effects of hyperventilation and mouth breathing on nitric oxide absorption

Nitric oxide (NO) is an exceptionally important compound with extensive respiratory functions, ranging from bronchial and vascular dilation (similar to CO2 in airways) to ciliary motion and antibacterial defense. From a biochemical viewpoint, NO can be a key chemical that suppresses pathogens in alveoli and airways.

Nasal and sinus cavities are the known major sites of NO production, followed by airway and alveolar compartments (Rolla et al, 2005). However, while many lung pathologies are characterized by increased levels of NO in exhaled air and airways, concentrations of NO are decreased in the airways of patients with cystic fibrosis (e.g., Grasemann et al, 2000; Grasemann & Ratjen, 2002; Keen et al, 2010). Furthermore, as the title of one medical study claims, *"Impaired lung diffusing capacity for nitric oxide and alveolar-capillary membrane conductance results in oxygen desaturation during exercise in patients with cystic fibrosis"* (Wheatley et al, 2011).

Hyperventilation, mouth breathing and tissue hypoxia are known factors that disrupt normal synthesis and absorption of nitric oxide. Let us consider the contributions of these effects.

The generation and absorption of increased levels of NO explains some of the benefits of nose breathing rather than mouth breathing (Scadding et al, 2007). Hence, habitual mouth breathing, or mouth breathing during sleep, is a factor that leads to reduced NO levels in the airways and arterial blood. This causes problems with infections in airways and reduced oxygen transport in the cardiovascular system.

Hyperventilation, apart from biochemical effects related to synthesis of NO, causes changes in the breathing patterns of people. During normal breathing at rest, healthy people have a natural period of no breathing (an automatic pause), after each exhalation. This pause is followed by relatively short and fast diaphragmatic inhalation that creates turbulent air flow allowing better absorption of NO generated in sinuses. The exhalation, immediately after this inhalation, is passive, slow and relaxed - allowing generation of nitric oxide in sinuses. Therefore, a normal breathing pattern favors generation and effective utilization of nasal NO, and nasal NO output in the healthy subjects is four-fold greater during inhalation when compared to exhalation (Törnberg et al, 2002).

In contrast, hyperventilation is characterized by an absence of the automatic pause and forceful exhalations that have turbulent air flow so it blows off most of the nitric oxide generated in the sinuses.

Important note about airway clearance techniques for cystic fibrosis

Conventional chest physiotherapy often includes forceful high-velocity coughing through the mouth with inhalations through the mouth. Such therapy involves losses in alveolar CO_2, reduced nasal nitric oxide absorption, and overcooling and drying of airways due to large flow of air (hyperventilation). Russian medical doctors practicing the Buteyko method suggest that all coughing should be done through the nose, while mucus or sputum should be gently removed when it comes out naturally and is located inside the mouth. The most effective methods to encourage airway clearance are correct breathing exercises and physical activity with strictly nasal breathing because they lead to higher levels of alveolar CO_2. Increased CO_2 improves oxygenation and perfusion of hypoxic cilia cells naturally leading to restoration of their primary functions. Furthermore, this approach does not cause production of new sputum due to adverse effects of overbreathing.

Humming and nitric oxide

Nasal levels of NO can be increased 15-fold during humming compared with quiet exhalation (e.g., Weitzberg & Lundberg, 2002). Furthermore, clinical evidence suggests, according to the title of one study, that *"Strong humming for one hour daily to terminate chronic rhinosinusitis in four days: a case report and hypothesis for action by stimulation of endogenous nasal nitric oxide production"* (Eby et al 2006). In this report, it was found that the morning after the first 1 hour humming session, *"the subject awoke with a clear nose and found himself breathing easily through his nose for the first time in over 1 month. During the following 4 days, CRS [chronic rhinosinusitis] symptoms slightly reoccurred, but with much less intensity each day. By humming 60-120 times four times per day (with a session at bedtime), CRS symptoms were essentially eliminated in 4 days."*

Leading Soviet physiologist Konstantin Buteyko, MD, PhD also suggested that humming has some health benefits. Note that humming during breathing retraining can have either positive or negative effects on alveolar CO_2 levels depending on the current breathing parameters and other factors, e.g., after meals versus on an empty stomach, posture, metabolic rate (exercise), and some others.

3.4 Nocturnal hypoxemia or nocturnal oxygen desaturation

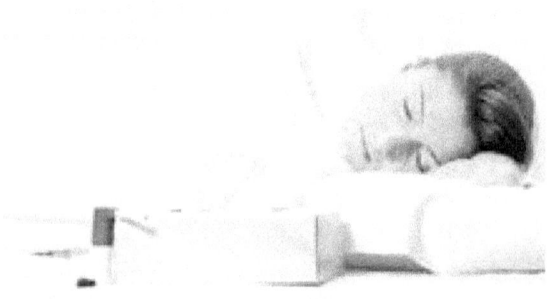

Another practical aspect related to breathing and cystic fibrosis is that for the overwhelming majority of CF patients, their worst hypoxemia (low blood oxygen saturation) and lowest body oxygenation take place during early morning hours or the last portion of the night sleep (Dancey et al, 2002; Frangolias & Wilcox, 2001; Salvatore & D'Andria, 2002; Young et al, 2011).

This effect is common in the sick, since early morning hours from about 4 to 7 am (as numerous medical studies have identified) have the highest mortality rates due to strokes, coronary artery spasms, acute asthma attacks, seizures and other exacerbations. Note that this effect of oxygen desaturation is even present in infants with cystic fibrosis (Villa et al, 2001).

While some researchers suggest that hypoventilation could be a factor that makes nocturnal oxygen desaturation possible, those studies that measured respiratory frequencies in CF patients reported their higher breathing rates. For example, the study conducted on infants (Villa et al, 2001) found that the average respiratory rate in infants with CF was 10 breaths/min higher than in normal infants. Furthermore, the authors suggested that, "... *Another predisposing factor for nocturnal desaturation was a high respiratory rate, an expression of possible lung impairment. Accordingly, subjects who had higher respiratory rates also had lower SaO2 values during sleep*" (Villa et al, 2001).

Hence, thoracic (or upper chest) breathing, when combined with hypoventilation and high respiratory rates, leads to abnormally low blood oxygenation values. These clinical findings indicate that abdominal breathing and slowing down the respiratory rates should be essential parts of breathing retraining in CF.

4. Can automatic breathing be retrained?

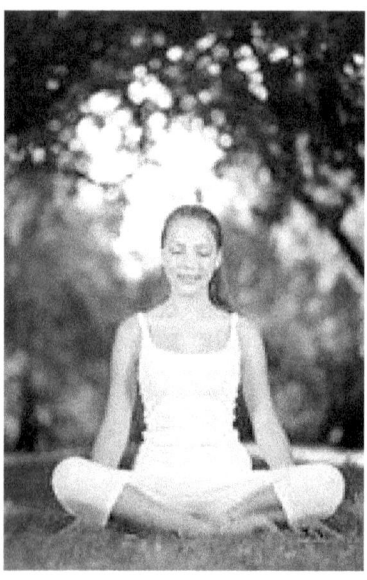

Chronic hyperventilation in CF at rest can have two explanations.

1. Chronic overbreathing can be the result of the disease and then we can declare that abnormal breathing has nothing to do with CF. Then we also need to assume that it is hard or impossible to change one's automatic breathing pattern back to the medical norm, and we are going to try to find other methods and techniques, apart from breathing retraining, to address the symptoms of CF.

2. The second approach is to assume that heavy breathing causes tissue hypoxia, CFTR expression and development of CF. Then we can apply all known therapies for cystic fibrosis (medication, digestive enzymes, physiotherapy, lifestyle changes related to diet, exercise, and so forth) and use breathing retraining as an additional or supplementary technique with the goal to change or normalize automatic or basal breathing in people with cystic fibrosis.

Which way to choose? Consider supporting medical evidence.

4.1 Hyperventilation provocation test

It is well known that the hyperventilation provocation test is a 100% specific test that readily provokes the main symptoms of angina pain, asthma, epilepsy, and panic attacks. For example, voluntary over-breathing in people with hypertension causes the heart attack, in asthmatics – the asthma attack, in epileptics – epilepsy seizures, etc. Here is a summary of some medical studies regarding different health conditions, number of patients investigated, and the percentage of patients who reproduced their specific health problem:
- coronary artery spasms (Nakao et al, 1997) 206 patients, 100% specific;
- bronchial asthma (Mojsoski & Pavicic, 1990) 90 patients, 100% specific;
- panic attacks (Bonn et al, 1984; Holt & Andrews, 1989; Nardi et al, 2000), 95% specific;
- epileptic absence seizures (Esquivel, 1991; Wirrel, 1996).

All these symptoms (chest pain, wheezing, seizures, etc.) can be expected since they are based on known laws of physiology related to oxygen and carbon dioxide changes (considered above).

It is also known that symptomatic application of reduced breathing decreases the severity of symptoms. For example, clinical experience of Russian Buteyko doctors testifies that most asthmatics can stop acute asthma attacks using a simple breathing exercise instead of using ventolin or other medication (Buteyko et al, 1968; Genina, 1982). The same breathing exercise can unblock the nose for people with sinusitis. Reduced breathing can stop most coronary artery spasms as well (Buteyko et al, 1965).

So we see from two different perspectives - hyperventilation provocation and intentionally reduced breathing - that purposeful, short-term changes in breathing patterns can have dramatic physiological effects. This raises the question "Can systematic breathing retraining permanently alter automatic breathing patterns to produce long-term positive effects"?

4.2 What are the effects of breathing training on people with CF?

Clinical trials of various breathing training techniques have so far been limited to the application of biofeedback assisted breathing retraining. The purpose has been to develop *diaphragmatic breathing using the pursed-lip breathing technique* (Delk et al, 1994) and *inspiratory muscle training* (e.g., de Jong et al, 2001; Enright et al, 2004).

During the first such study, the experimental subjects "*underwent eight sessions of pneumographic or strain-gauge feedback from the abdominal muscles and electromyogram feedback from accessory respiratory muscles to assist in learning diaphragmatic and pursed-lips breathing maneuvers*" (Delk et al, 1994). They experienced a 38 percent (clinically significant) increase in FEF25; 50; and 75% after 4 weeks of diaphragmatic breathing. There were no significant changes (3%) in the control group. There was also a 29% improvement in FVC (significant) for the experimental group. The FVC percent change in the control group was 8% (insignificant).

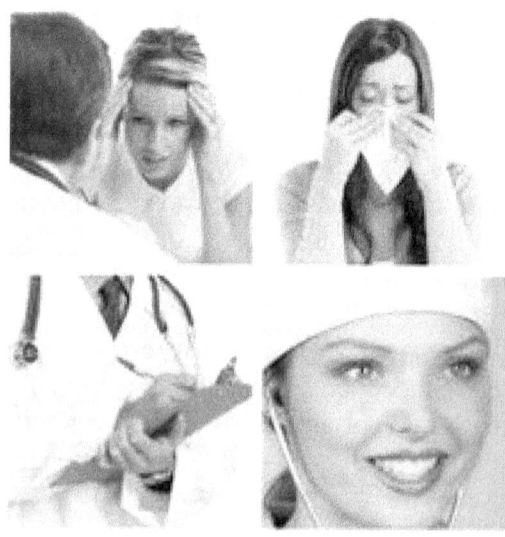

One clinical trial of *inspiratory muscle training* found that low-intensity inspiratory-threshold loading (at the level of 40% of maximum inspiratory pressure) produced an increased inspiratory-muscle endurance in patients with CF (de Jong et al, 2001). However, since this trial did not intend to address problems with chest breathing and low alveolar CO_2, there were no changes in pulmonary function tests.

Another inspiratory muscle training trial found improved lung function and exercise capacity in adults with cystic fibrosis (Enright et al, 2004). The effect was probably due to two factors: higher training intensity (80% of maximal inspiratory effort) and improved basal breathing patterns. This may be because the instructions for all respiratory trainers (Powerbreathe, Ultrabreathe, etc.) suggest that exhalations should be slow and relaxed. It is very likely that if the inhaled air has higher CO_2 content, as is the case with some breathing devices, breathing training can provide double benefits: improved strength of respiratory muscles; and improved automatic breathing patterns after the breathing session. This would lead to lasting biochemical effects related to improved cell oxygenation.

4.3 Clinical trials of the Buteyko breathing technique

The Buteyko breathing method is (also known as the Buteyko method or Buteyko breathing technique) is a system of activities that include breathing exercises and lifestyle changes. The program of lifestyle changes in the Buteyko method is similar to hatha yoga, but it has more science behind it. The goal of the technique is to normalize one's automatic or unconscious breathing pattern (learn how to breathe in accordance with medical norms 24/7). This method was created by Doctor Konstantin Buteyko.

There were 6 Western randomized clinical trials of the Buteyko breathing technique on subjects with asthma - another health condition that involves pathological changes in the lungs. All these trials found that the control groups could significantly reduce their short-term bronchodilator use by up to 70-90% and steroid use by about 50% in 3-6 months. But there were no changes in abnormal lung function results.

Furthermore, while most subjects with asthma had improvements in various tested parameters (less medication, better quality of life, reduced symptom score, and reduced frequency of infections), there were a few people who got worse at the end of these trials. This fact indicates that there are certain hidden factors that can also influence automatic breathing patterns, and, for some people, these hidden factors can play a crucial role in their long-term respiratory changes.

The central question, however, in relation to all these trials of the Buteyko method is this: Did the control group achieve **normal breathing parameters**? This question is very important because Dr. Konstantin Buteyko made 2 essential physiological claims in relation to many chronic diseases, asthma and CF included:
1). Sick people suffer from alveolar hypocapnia (lack of CO_2) caused by chronic hyperventilation at rest
2) If they normalize their breathing, their symptoms and diseases are going to disappear.

Available data suggests that the control groups during these 6 clinical trials did not achieve the medical norm (6 L/min, 10-12 breaths/min, 500-600 ml for tidal volume, 40 mm Hg for alveolar CO2m and so forth). What were the final breathing parameters in these 6 Western trials? The asthmatics with the best results started with about 12 L/min and finished with about 9 L/min. Hence, they got only half way to the medical norm.

But Dr. Buteyko did not claim that partial breathing normalization can cure asthma. Furthermore, doctor Buteyko established different norms for breathing, such as 4 L/min, 8 breaths/min, 500 ml for tidal volume (amount of air for one breath), and about 46 mm Hg for alveolar CO_2. His physiological requirement to cure asthma is to slow breathing down to about 4 L/min for minute ventilation and 46 mm Hg for alveolar CO_2 pressure.

Therefore, we can conclude that these clinical trials tested the abilities of Buteyko breathing practitioners to reduce symptoms and

Cystic Fibrosis

medication in asthma. Meanwhile, the trials did not address the key physiological statements proposed by Dr. Buteyko in relation to asthma.

5. Body oxygen test, breathing patterns, morning CP

5.1 How to Measure Body Oxygen Level (DIY Test)

Sit down and rest for 5-7 minutes. Completely relax all your muscles, including the breathing muscles. This relaxation produces natural spontaneous exhalation (breathing out). Pinch your nose closed at the end of this exhalation and count your BHT (breath holding time) in seconds. Keep the nose pinched until you experience the first desire to breathe. Practice shows that this first desire appears together with an involuntary push of the diaphragm or swallowing movement in the throat. (Your body warns you, "Enough!") If you release the nose and start breathing at this time, you can resume your usual breathing pattern (in the same way as you were breathing prior to the test).

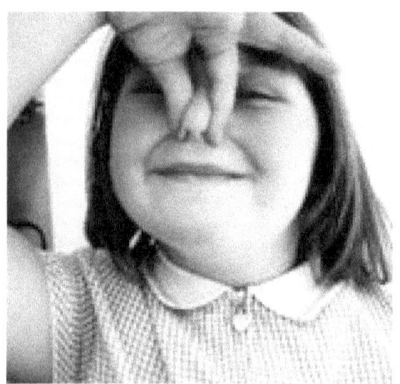

Do not extend breath holding too long trying to increase the control pause. You should not gasp for air or open your mouth when you release your nose. The test should be easy and not cause you any stress. This breath holding time test should not interfere with your breathing, as shown here:

Cystic Fibrosis

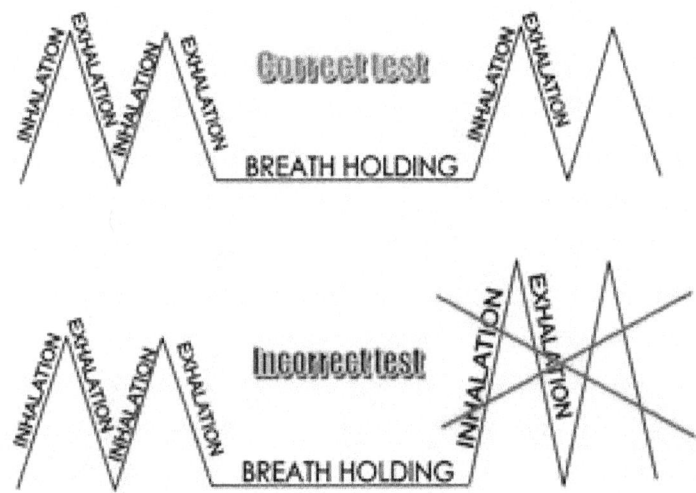

Warning. Some, not all, people with heart disease, migraine headaches, and panic attacks may experience negative symptoms minutes later after this light version of the test. If this happens, they should temporary avoid this test until they get higher CP.

What about usual body oxygen numbers, CP norms and CP of sick and healthy people?

"If a person breath-holds after a normal exhalation, it takes about 40 seconds before breathing commences" From the textbook "Essentials of exercise physiology" McArdle W.D., Katch F.I., Katch V.L. (2nd edition); Lippincott, Williams and Wilkins, London 2000, p.252.

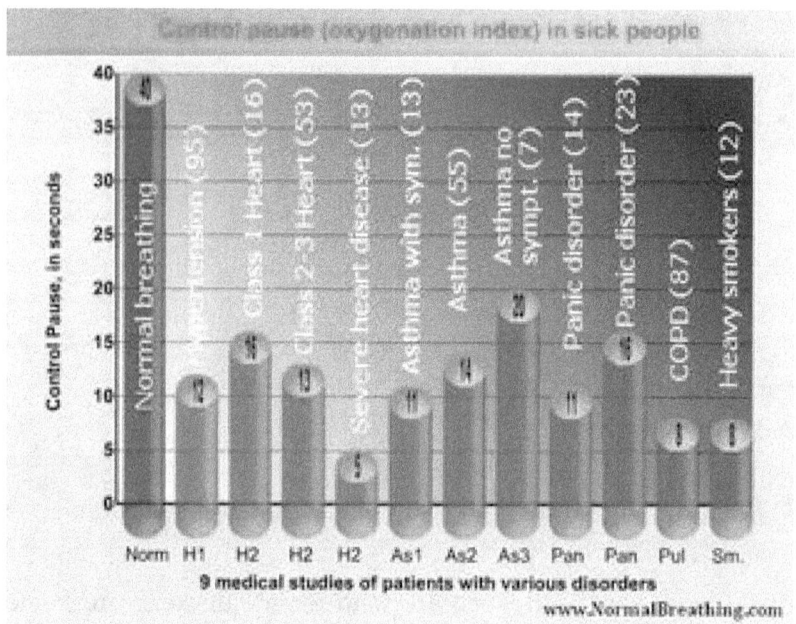

Results of Western medical and physiological research studies are summarized in these 2 Tables:

- CP (body oxygen test) in sick people (13 medical studies; less than 20 s) - http://www.normalbreathing.com/index-CP-sick.php

- CP (body oxygen test) in healthy people (24 references; about 20-30 s now; about 40-50 s some 80-100 years ago) - http://www.normalbreathing.com/index-CP-normals.php

Now we know that people with mild forms of chronic diseases have about 15 seconds for the body oxygen test. My experience with thousands of sick people suggests exactly the same. Doctor Buteyko and his medical colleagues tested more than a hundred thousand patients.

Here is a short summary of typical results for the body oxygen test:

1-10 s - severely sick, critically and terminally ill patients, usually hospitalized.

10-20 s - sick patients with numerous complaints and, often, on daily medication.

20-30 s - people with average health and usually without serious chronic health problems.

40-60 s - very good health.

Over 60 s - ideal health, when many modern diseases are virtually impossible.

5.2 Breathing patterns and body oxygenation

Now we need to find the link between the body oxygen test results and basal or automatic breathing patters. For example, if we consider healthy people with normal breathing parameters (or the normal breathing pattern: 6 L/min, 10-12 breaths per minute, 10-12 breaths/min at rest while sitting), they have about 35-40 seconds for the body oxygen test.

What about people with low CP? If you visit the Homepage of www.NormalBreathing.com, you can see a large Table with about 50 medical studies that measured minute ventilation in sick people, In average, sick people breathe about 12-18 L/min or 2-3 times more than the medical norm. What did we find about their body oxygen test results? Their body O2 content is about 2-3 times less than the norm. Dr. Buteyko tested thousands of sick and healthy people in his laboratory and he found that there is a nearly linear relationship between minute ventilation and the CP.

If you breathe twice the norm, your CP will be 2 times less than the norm or about 20 seconds. If you breathe for 4 people, your CP is about 10 seconds only. These ideas are reflected on the following graph that represents parameters of 4 automatic breathing patterns.

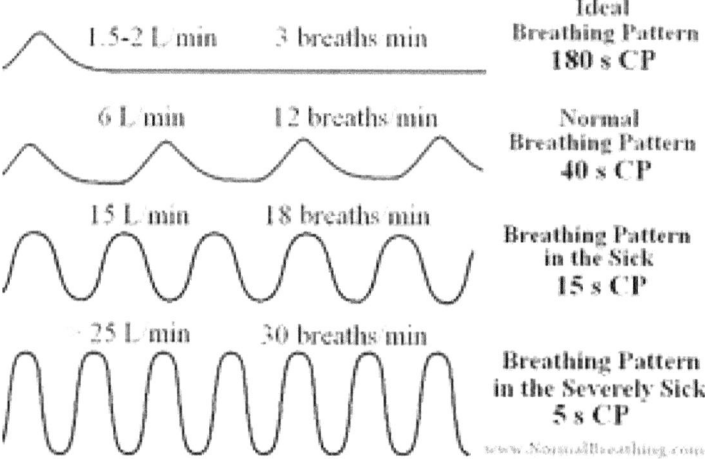

5.3. Morning CP: your main health test

Physiological, medical and epidemiological studies have clearly shown that people with severe forms of heart disease, asthma, COPD, epilepsy, and many other conditions are most likely to die during early morning hours (4-7 am), when their breathing is the heaviest, body oxygenation is critically low, and the CP is the shortest (about 5 seconds or less). You can investigate relevant medical quotes and observations of western medical doctors on the webpage "Morning Hyperventilation" (www.normalbreathing.com/index- MorningHV.php) or by watching my YouTube video-clip "Sleep Heavy Breathing Effect" (http://www.youtube.com/watch?v=Vj_8J8BcTi8).

Most people also experience the shortest CPs during early morning hours and feel worst in the morning after waking up. Practical observations of Buteyko breathing teachers have confirmed that, indeed, in most people, up to 80% or more, their CPs significantly drops (up to 3-7 seconds or even more) during the night.

There are many causes that contribute to this Morning Hyperventilation effect. However, the very first aim for each person is to identify the presence and extent of this problem. How? Measure your CP immediately after waking up in the morning. As soon as you open your eyes, before getting out of the bed, do the stress-free breath holding time test. Have a ticking or other clock or watch nearby to help you define your breathing rate during last hours of sleep.

The MCP (morning control pause) is the most important parameter of your physiological health.

You can record this number in your daily log for breathing exercises that can be downloaded from NormalBreathing.com (Free Downloads Section).

Dr. Artour Rakhimov

6. Clinical experience of Russian doctors in relation to cystic fibrosis

Two large groups of Russian MDs (hundreds of doctors) have developed and applied two different breathing therapies (the Buteyko breathing technique and Frolov breathing device therapy) for CF and found that it is possible to reverse symptoms of cystic fibrosis with improved basal breathing. Furthermore, based on their clinical experience, Buteyko doctors suggested the following relationships between respiratory parameters, prognosis, stages, life expectancy and symptoms of CF patients (see explanations below).

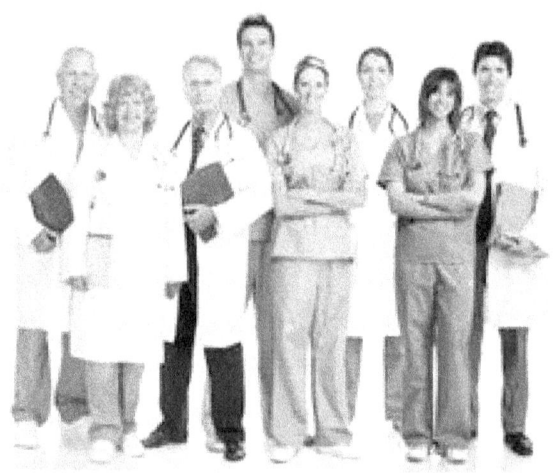

Stages, life expectancy and prognosis for cystic fibrosis patients and their respiratory parameters

Cystic Fibrosis

CP range	Stages of the disease	Usual life expectancy	Symptoms and prognosis
1-5 seconds	End-stage disease	Some months	Quickly developing and severe problems with lungs (possible cor pulmonale), chronic indigestion, etc.
6-10 s	Clinical stage (hospitalization or palliative care is required)	Less than 1-2 years	Worsened health state with progressive respiratory deterioration: bronchitis and bronchiolitis transform into bronchiectasis; possible complications include hemoptysis and pneumothorax.
11-20 s	Moderate individual symptoms	Up to 30-40 years	A typical patient with classical symptoms of mild cystic fibrosis including chronic infections, poor exercise tolerance, inflammation, GI symptoms,...
20-40 s	Initial stage of the disease	Up to 40-60 years	Mild GI symptoms; slight deterioration in lung function tests
over 40 s 24/7	Normal health	Normal	No symptoms; normal life expectancy

*CP (Control Pause or body oxygen test) test measures the duration of **stress-free** breath holding done **after** usual exhalation. It is also called the body oxygen test.*

Clinical observations of these MDs resulted in the following suggestions. The progress of cystic fibrosis and worsened respiratory and digestive symptoms are possible only in conditions of chronic hyperventilation and/or ineffective chest breathing leading to cell hypoxia. The prognosis and life expectancy in these patients depends on the degree of alveolar hyperventilation.

They discovered that damage to lungs, sinuses, pancreas, liver, intestines, and sex organs in cystic fibrosis is proportional to the degree of respiratory abnormalities, while a complete clinical remission in patients with cystic fibrosis takes place in cases of breathing normalization (Dr. Buteyko's norms). Hence, they claim that patients with cystic fibrosis have an excellent prognosis and normal life expectancy if they can normalize their automatic breathing patterns.

I also had students with cystic fibrosis. Their CP test results were in agreement with the Table. The only significance difference that I noticed in relation to people with cystic fibrosis was that their CP progress was about twice slower for the same amount of efforts in comparison with other typical students. For example, if there are two similar students to learn breathing retraining, and one has mild asthma and another one cystic fibrosis, then the person with asthma will require about 2-3 weeks to get up to 25 s for the morning CP and be free from asthma medication (i.e., asthma inhalers or bronchodilators) and main symptoms of asthma. However, the person with cystic fibrosis requires about 2 times more time or about 4-6 weeks to get to the same CP level. Therefore, presence of the defective gene make the progress slower, but does not prevent them from getting great health.

That makes sense since physiological changes and damage to the human organism due to cystic fibrosis involves not only lungs, but also digestive organs. People with cystic fibrosis just require a little bit more efforts in their journeys to better health.

7. Breathing exercises for higher CP

Practice show that when a person has low CP, the CP has a tendency to gradually become smaller and smaller. That explains why sick people generally become sicker and sicker. Restoration of normal breathing (or breathing normalization) requires 2 types of activities: **breathing exercises** that are able to increase body oxygenation and **lifestyle changes** that leads to slower and easier breathing, and higher CPs.

There are over 15 different breathing techniques and methods that has been used and applied by health practitioners and doctors in various situations, cystic fibrosis included.

7.1 Buteyko breathing method

The Buteyko Breathing Technique (also known as the Buteyko method or Buteyko breathing method) is the most advanced system in relation to lifestyle changes. It has 6 excellent Western clinical trials on asthma that are considered in Section 4.3 above.

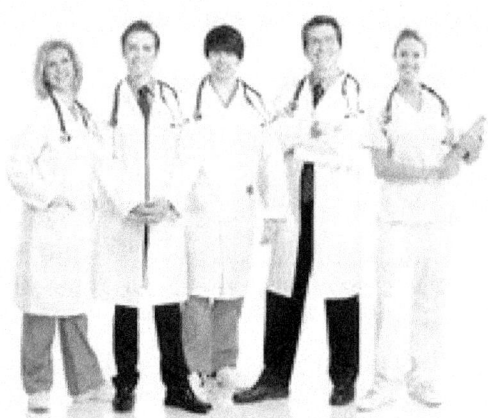

Another additional advantage of the Buteyko method is that it uses a highly sensitive and simple body oxygen test (the Buteyko Control Pause) to monitor the progress in breathing retraining and effects of lifestyle changes. (The Buteyko program related to lifestyle changes are analyzed in the next Chapter.)

However, the Buteyko breathing exercises are not the most effective ones, especially for people who have problems with lungs. Buteyko exercises are also not so easy to learn without a Buteyko breathing practitioner. The better option in relation to breathing exercises and faster health recovery is to use breathing devices.

7.2 Frolov breathing device

The Frolov breathing device (or Frolov respiration training device) is a modern respiratory training device. It was invented by Vladimir Fedorovich Frolov and Eugene Fedorovich Kustov in the 1990's. Numerous Russian clinical trials and approbations have found that the Frolov device is safe and effective medical tool to reduce symptoms and medication for various health problems (including asthma, bronchitis, COPD, emphysema, hypertension, angina pectoris, sinusitis, diabetes, arthritis, seizures, sleep apnea, and many other conditions).

In Russia, the Frolov breathing device can be bought in pharmacies and hundreds of Russian MDs or family physicians prescribe the Frolov breathing device to their patients so that they can buy and use it.

Apart from two patents in the USSR and Russia, the Frolov respiration device was patented in the USA - Patent Number 5,755,640 (here is a PDF file: 1998 USA Frolov Device Patent - http://www.normalbreathing.com/downloads/US5755640-frolov-device-patent.pdf). In the USA, since 2000 the Frolov breathing device was officially approved by the US FDA (Food and Drug Administration) as a Class 2 medical device (Frolov FDA's approval - http://www.accessdata.fda.gov/cdrh_docs/pdf/k992256.pdf).

When following the holistic health restoration program, based on Dr KP Buteyko discoveries in relation to lifestyle changes and the general goal of breathing training (breathe less and slower 24/7), breathing sessions with the Frolov device deliver the fastest growth in body oxygen content (the control pause - see the test below) in comparison with other popular techniques.

7.3 Amazing DIY breathing device

The [Amazing DIY Breathing Device](http://www.normalbreathing.com/book-DIY-breathing-device.php) is a prototype of the Frolov device. The Amazing DIY breathing device produces comparable or even better results in comparison with the Frolov device, if you are a mildly handy person.

Generally, the Frolov device is an idea tool for people with less than 15 s CP and especially those people who suffer from any problems with lungs, such as asthma, bronchitis and cystic fibrosis. However, when the CP gets higher, the exhalation becomes also longer and the stimulating effect on the lungs and other body organs (due to changes in air pressure due to inhalations and exhalations) becomes smaller.

The Amazing DIY breathing device solves this problem. When a person gets up to 20-25 seconds for the current CP, he or she can construct the device with much larger resistance. More challenging device increases efficiency of the breathing sessions and leads to higher CP after the session.

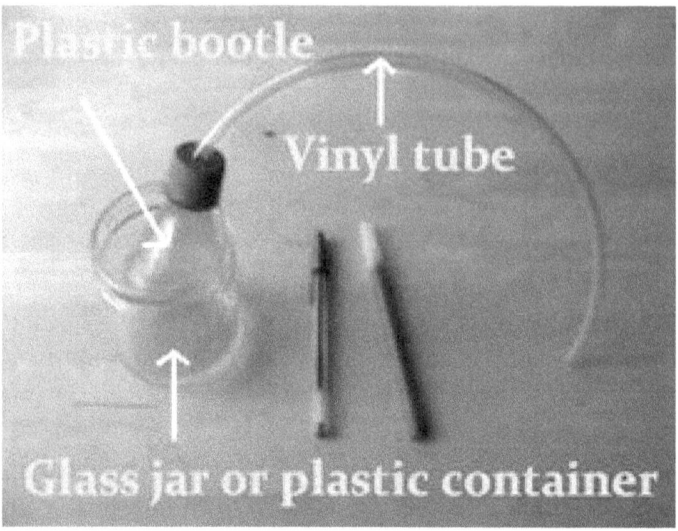

7.4 Breathing exercises for people with cystic fibrosis

If we compare the effects of various breathing exercises, the Frolov breathing device and the Amazing DIY breathing device produce better results than the Buteyko breathing exercises. This is especially true for people with lung pathologies, since breathing devices have effects on training of inspiratory and expiratory muscles, lymphatic nodes located beneath the diaphragm and simplicity of practice (no need for a breathing teacher - which is necessary with the Buteyko method).

The average increase in body oxygen test results for people with lung pathologies is about 50-70% higher for suitable breathing devices in comparison with the Buteyko breathing exercise session of the same duration.

Therefore, in my view, the most advanced system of breathing retraining for people with less than 20 seconds for the body oxygen test and for most people with moderate and severe cystic fibrosis includes the use of breathing devices that:
- create resistance to breathing during inhalations and exhalations
- trap exhaled air so that to increase CO_2 levels in the lungs

- use abdominal breathing with large amplitudes and muscular relaxation.

Additional factors for more effective breathing exercises with breathing devices involve the use of essential oils and other herbs, and **use of warm water** (to prevent inflammation of airways due to cold air during breathing exercises) or warmed up devices to prevent overcooling of airways. Correction of lifestyle factors is very important, and they depend on health states and symptoms of the students.

7.5 Oxygen Remedy online webinars

www.OxygenRemedy.org is probably the most comprehensive breathing retraining course that is taught by me. There are 17 online webinar lessons as well as support provided by Richard Geller (the main organizer of Oxygen Remedy online webinars). This course uses the most advanced breathing exercises and methods related to lifestyle changes

8. Lifestyle program for high body oxygen in CF

The following lifestyle adjustments are intended to prevent hyperventilation, mouth breathing, chest breathing, or their combinations in order to keep breathing light and the body oxygen levels as high as possible.

8.1 Morning CP is the main health parameter in cystic fibrosis

During the night we do not control our breathing. For most people breathing is heaviest between about 3 and 6 am. The effect is very common in cystic fibrosis, and mainstream medicine call it "nocturnal hypoxemia" (as discussed above). Hence, in people with CF, the CP is lowest during these early morning hours. Remember: **severely sick people are most likely to have acute episodes or attacks, or even die during early morning hours (4-7 am), when their breathing is heaviest and body oxygenation lowest. This is true for people with cystic fibrosis, heart disease, stroke, COPD, asthma, epilepsy and many other conditions.**

In cystic fibrosis, the main damage to the body (generation of free radicals, oxidative stress, increased inflammation and infections) takes place during early morning hours when the person has his or her lowest CP. Hence, the morning CP is the main parameter of health in CF as well.

Each morning, as soon you wake up, while you are still in bed, you should measure your morning CP. This should be done immediately after you open your eyes. Why? Just 5-10 minutes later your breathing parameters can be different and the crucial information about your breathing during the last hours of sleep can be lost. If you cannot do this breath-holding test because of contraindications (high blood pressure, panic attacks, and so forth), measure your heart rate during 1 minute and record it in your daily log.

Cystic Fibrosis

Your changes in morning CP numbers will be used later for finding the hidden causes of the problem with morning hyperventilation (discussed below). In addition, to find out the degree of this problem, you should also measure the evening CP every night, just before going to sleep. This will indicate the progress achieved during that particular day.

The morning CP is not just a test. It also provides you with energy and reminds you about your commitment to breathe less.

After several days of measurements, there are many numbers - daily, evening and morning CPs. Then the goal is to find out the emerging pattern related to personal circadian CP changes. Is the morning CP much smaller than the previous evening CP? By how much?

Experience shows that the overwhelming majority of people with CF have a large CP drop (5 s or more) during the night. For some people, the drop is even more drastic.

Practicing breathing exercises and many other useful activities during the course of the day gradually restores the CO_2 level and the CP back to their usual daily values. However, during the next night, the pattern is repeated again: good daytime values followed by a morning CP drop.

Would the morning CP improve if breathing exercises and common sense activities were practiced for several weeks? The experience of Buteyko breathing method practitioners shows that usually it will. But it is physiologically obvious that low morning CP would be the greatest factor impeding the general CP progress and health restoration.

It would make sense, therefore, to address the problem directly and analyze the factors that contribute to low morning CP. Some of these factors, the most common ones, are discussed below. But you have to be your own detective to reveal your personal factors that make your morning CP low. And you need to investigate, analyze and correct your health-related factors until your morning CP is about the same as your evening CP.

8.2 Sleeping positions

Medical research (over 20 studies) testifies to the adverse effects of supine sleeping on different groups of adults. Scientific studies have found that sleeping on the back leads to higher incidence of sleep paralysis (with terrifying hallucinations), stroke, asthma, increased airway resistance (since CO2 is a natural bronchodilator), and sleep apnea episodes. Several studies found lowered blood oxygenation in people who sleep on their backs. These abstracts are quoted in Module 6-B: Best Sleep Positions - http://www.normalbreathing.com/l-6-best-sleep-positions.php

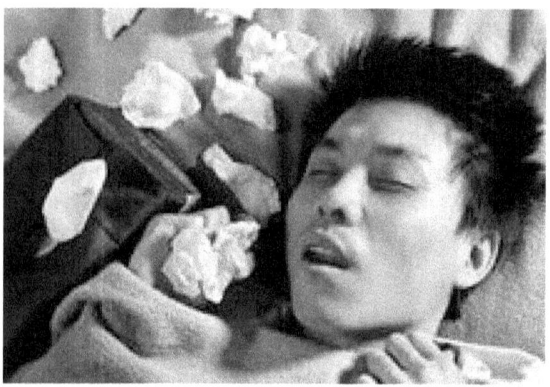

If you are uncertain about this, do your personal testing. Measure your body oxygen level (the CP test) after resting in different sleeping positions. Your body oxygen level, according to all available medical evidence, is the best and simplest known DIY test for personal health. The CP reflects your stress-free breath-holding time after your usual exhalation. You can use an electrical clock with elimination showing seconds or a ticking mechanical clock so that there is no need to turn the light on during the night. Note that you should spend about 10-15 minutes in each position in order to achieve a stable metabolism before you measure your CP.

Sleeping on the back is worst and causes lowest body oxygenation since our breathing is unrestricted: our belly and chest muscles can move without any restrictions. As a result, sleeping on one's back

Cystic Fibrosis

intensifies breathing and leads to the appearance of an ineffective, heavy, and/or irregular breathing pattern.

For many sick people, sleeping on the back means about twice as much breathing and a corresponding CP drop (almost 2 times less). This often causes acute symptoms during the early morning hours and death in severely sick people. Hence, Dr. Buteyko, his medical colleagues, and their numerous patients have used a variety of techniques how to prevent sleeping on the back.

8.3 Methods to prevent back sleeping

Take a sock and wrap it around the middle of a belt making a knot. The belt can be positioned around the middle of the chest with the knot on your back. The knot should be big enough to prevent you from sleeping on your back. Since the knot is soft, it shouldn't wake you up.

Here in another popular solution. Take a double layer (strip) of bed linen about 2 m long and 20-30 cm wide. Wrap it around yourself, make two knots on your chest and move them around to your back. A simple scarf can be also used.

The experience of Buteyko breathing teachers shows that sleeping on the back is the sign of low CP. This problem is present when the CP is about 20 s or less. Once your morning CP is over 25 s, you are very unlikely to sleep on your back at all and there is no need to use any of these techniques.

8.4 Sleeping in a sitting position: highest body oxygen results

The health of any person with cystic fibrosis will be much better if he or she can learn how to sleep in a sitting position. (If your health really matters to you, go for it.) Dr. Buteyko and his colleagues agree that sitting is the best sleeping position for human beings. The CP remains almost unchanged. Sleeping sitting requires a solid strong chair, head-neck support, support for elbows (to relax the arms) and nearly vertical position of the torso (avoiding reclining). It takes several days to adapt to it. If your sleep gets much shorter because of higher CPs and sleeping upright (a great result), you may need to take a short during the day. But avoid daytime sleep in the horizontal position.

8.5 Nose breathing 24/7

Nose breathing 24/7 is a must for people with cystic fibrosis. Mouth breathing may occur in the following situations: during daytime due to a blocked nose, during sleep at night, and during physical exercise.

Unblock the Nose in 1-2 min (Breathing Exercise)

Most patients with cystic fibrosis, according to the clinical experience of Russian Buteyko doctors, could unblock the blocked nose and resume their nasal breathing in about one-two minutes naturally. This remedy also works for people with chronic sinusitis and can be applied during the night as well (see below).

How to do the exercise to unblock the nose

Pinch your nose. Walk fast with your blocked nose pinched and your mouth closed all the time. You will be able to take around 15-25 steps. While walking, you should hold your breath until you feel a strong urge to breathe. Then sit down with your spine totally straight and focus on your breath. After you release your nose, resume your usual breathing and keep the mouth closed. Hence, instead of taking a big inhalation, take a smaller inhale and then relax all muscles for exhalation, especially upper chest and other respiratory muscles. Make another (smaller) inhale and again relax.

Cystic Fibrosis

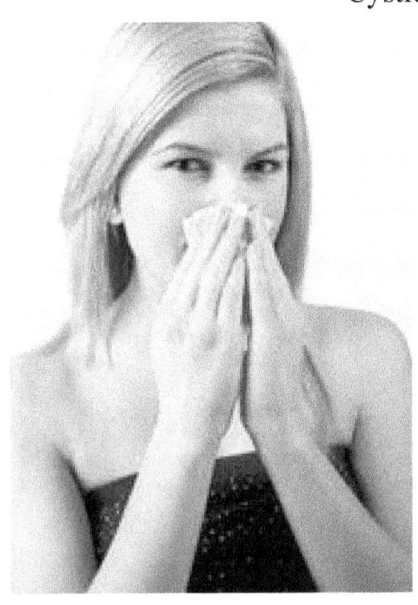

With each inhalation, practice this reduced or shallow breathing while remaining relaxed. Your main goal is to maintain air hunger for about 2-3 min with total relaxation of body muscles. The breathing can be frequent during this reduced breathing exercise but this is normal. If later your breathing becomes heavy (deep and/or fast), your nose will get blocked again. Then you can repeat this exercise.

Steps to follow during night sleep to unblock the nose

Lie on your left side or chest and relax all your muscles. Pinch your nose and follow the above instructions related to breath holding and reduced breathing to get quick relief. If your nose gets blocked again and again, you should increase your body oxygenation up to 20 s using breath work (see below).

How to tape your mouth at night to prevent mouth breathing

For mouth taping at night, one needs a surgical tape and cream to prevent the tape sticking. Both can be bought in the pharmacy. Micropore (or 3M) and vaseline are popular choices. First, put a small amount of cream on the lips so that it is easy to remove the tape in the morning. Then take a small piece of tape and stick it in the middle, vertically, across the closed mouth. Some students prefer to put it horizontally, but a small piece in the middle is sufficient. If you are afraid to "seal" your mouth completely, tape only one half of the mouth leaving space for emergency breathing.

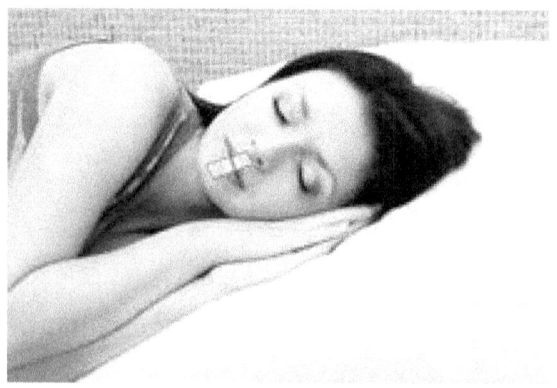

In 2006 one of my Buteyko breathing method colleagues, Dr. James Oliver, a GP from England and former president of the BBA (Buteyko Breathing Association) in the UK, made a presentation to the British Thoracic Society. He showed the safety of mouth taping based on thousands of cases both in Russia and in the west.

Mouth taping at night to stop mouth breathing normally should be a temporary measure. When your CP is above 20 s in the morning, mouth taping is not necessary.

Nose breathing during exercise

Nasal breathing during physical exercise is absolutely necessary for people with cystic fibrosis due to its numerous benefits. Generally, people with less than 20 s for the current CP cannot do any vigorous exercise with nose breathing only (in and out). Hence, it is necessary to slow down and do lighter forms of exercise until the CP is more than 20 s.

Breathing exercises with breathing devices are excellent options to boost the CP. This boost will enable you to get involved in physical activity since, in the long run, physical exercise is the key factor that will keep your CP high.

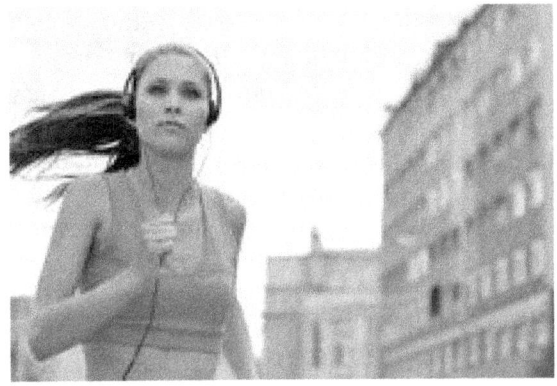

At more than 40 s morning CP, people enjoy and crave physical activity. Joining a local running club or training with other sport groups (basketball, soccer, cross-country skiing, and so forth) are excellent ways to maintain high CP.

8.6 Key physical activity factors that improve cell oxygen levels

- **Nasal breathing:** All physical activity should be done with nose breathing (inhalations and exhalations). This leads to increased use of CO2 and NO (nitric oxide) for the body cells, reduced heart rate for the same intensity of exercise, better oxygen transport, increased aerobic metabolism, and decreased lactic acid production. (See Effects of Exercise on the Respiratory System - http://www.normalbreathing.com/c-effects-of-exercise-on-the-respiratory-system.php for further details.) If you have a low level of fitness and decide to start jogging, it should be done very gradually. Follow the ideas related to gradual increase in physical activity: Benefits of Running - http://www.normalbreathing.com/benefits-of-running.php
- **Duration of physical activity**: The longer the exercise session, the stronger its impact.
- **Intensity or speed**: Generally, at lower CPs (less than 25-30 s), the most effective exercise is one that is done with maximum intensity,

but with nasal breathing all the time. At higher CPs (over 30 s), breathing control after exercise becomes an important factor that determines its maximum usefulness.
- **Perspiration**: Sweating removes numerous toxic and waste products assisting the GI tract, liver, kidneys and other body organs. Dr. Buteyko suggested that it is necessary for good health to sweat every day.
- **Shaking or mechanical vibrations of the whole body:** Each step, as during running or jogging, stimulates the lymphatic system and promotes the removal of waste products (which are develop during so called "physical diseases").

8.7 List of common factors for higher morning CP

1. If you find that your mouth is dry in the morning, use the mouth taping technique.

2. Prevent supine sleep using one of the methods described above.

3. Do more physical activity during the day, but with constant nasal breathing only (both in and out). Even sick people (when the CP is less than 20 s) benefit from such exercise, despite the fact that they may only be able to walk (not run) with nasal breathing.

4. Ensure that you sweat sufficiently (perspiration) and that your body vibrates (mechanical vibrations as when running) for at least 20-30 min every day (e.g., during physical exercise).

5. Avoid big meals late at night: have your supper at about 4 or 5 pm and eat a small snack later (at about 9 pm), only if you get really hungry.

6. Ensure excellent air quality in the place where you sleep (no carpets; open windows or use an air ionizer).

7. Do not overheat yourself at night (choose temperature, blanket, and other parameters to feel just comfortable or, if your CP is more than 20 s, even slightly on the cold side).

8. Follow 2 simple sleep rules: go to sleep only when you are really sleepy (not at a certain time) and do not stay in bed after you wake up in the morning.

9. Add those nutrients to your diet that could be missing in your body (fish oil for EFAs, Mg, Ca, Zn) since any deficiency will worsen your CP, quality of sleep, and morning health parameters.

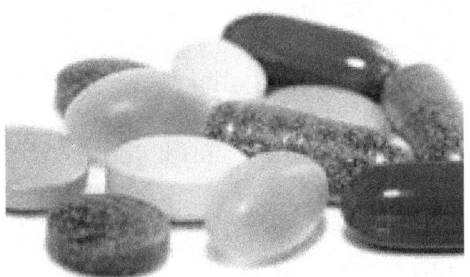

8.8 Diet and meals

This is the area where mainstream medicine has achieved many positive advances in helping people with CF through the use of digestive enzymes and other supplements. There are, however, additional ideas, such as food combining, use of a 3-day test to define nutritional deficiencies, better chewing, etc. that will help to achieve better GI flora and digestion. There are separate web pages on NormalBreathing.com devoted to these topics.

Organic food and purified water (e.g., reverse osmosis) will improve GI health in people with cystic fibrosis. Dr. Buteyko suggested that using sea salt is beneficial for patients with lung conditions. While numerous Western medical studies have found that salt causes problems for various health problems, this research has been focused on table salt (highly refined mineral salt). There is no scientific evidence of negative health effects from sea salt.

8.9 Focal infections

Certain health problems, such as focal infections, prevent breathing normalization. Hence, they require additional medical attention. Among the most common focal infections are:
- cavities in teeth (dental caries)
- degenerated tonsils causing frequent tonsillar infections
- foot mycosis (athlete's foot fungal infection)
- intestinal parasites (e.g., helminths)

All of them are analyzed on the web page Buteyko Focal Infections - http://www.normalbreathing.com/l-buteyko-focal-infections.php.
Root canals and mercury fillings often have nearly the same negative contribution to chronic diseases as these focal infections. There is no place in the mouth of the person with cystic fibrosis for root canals and mercury amalgam fillings.

8.10 Earthing: Get Grounded to Earth

Electrical grounding (also known as "Earthing") is an additional positive factor to increase body O2. It provides free electrons for the human body. Many students found this technique beneficial since it helps to slow down breathing and increase one's CP (often by 2 or more seconds). In a long run, Earthing can increase one's CP by up to 7-10 seconds. For many sick people, it is a crucial factor that helps them to break through 20, and later 30 and 40 s for the morning CP. Earthing can counteract inflammation, psychological stress, muscle pain, back pain and other problems. For an average person with cystic fibrosis, Earthing can accelerate their CP progress up to 50-200%. Many students are unable to increase their CP without Earthing due to excessive inflammation in airways and GI tract.

The human body has a tendency to accumulate positive electrical charge (up to many 100 or 1,000s Volts), while Earth has a slightly negative charge (or excess of electrons). Since many antioxidants, like vitamin C, are able to disactivate free radicals by donating to them electrons, Earthing can produce a similar effect as antioxidants.

The technique can be used for some part of the day or during sleep. Sleep grounding is the suggested method especially for those people who have low morning CP. One can make simple DIY devices for using Earthing during sleep. The same or similar devices can be applied during daytime.

As a simplest solution, you can get electrically connected (or grounded) with Earth using copper cables that can be found in electrical stores. One end of this cable can be attached to plumbing tubes and another to a small piece of copper that you can keep in your socks (on your feet) during sleep. You can find more ideas, suggestions, and links on this web page: Earthing – (http://www.normalbreathing.com/e/earthing.php) and How to ground yourself – (http://www.normalbreathing.com/e/how-to-ground-yourself.php).

8.11 No acute HV (hyperventilation)

It is important to prevent acute episodes of hyperventilation that can occur due to bouts of coughing, yawning, sneezing, and other activities accompanied by CO_2 losses. There are special breathing exercises and other techniques that can be found on web pages of NormalBreathing.com.

8.12 Additional factors

There are many other situational factors that can lead either to abnormal breathing and chronic hyperventilation or to easier breathing and higher body oxygen levels. For example, swaddling infants is beneficial because it increases alveolar CO_2 and prevents thoracic breathing. Correct posture aids abdominal breathing, while slouching leads to chest breathing and hypoxemia.

Poor air quality (e.g., carpets and books in bedrooms) drastically worsens the state of the airways and lungs causing hyperventilation. Hence, there is no place for carpets in the bedroom of a person with cystic fibrosis.

Similarly, any allergic trigger will worsen breathing. Hence, avoidance of allergies is important for breathing normalization and desensitization of the immune system.

Taking cold showers (while following several crucial rules and requirements developed by Buteyko doctors e.g., with more than 20 s CP), is exceptionally beneficial for people with cystic fibrosis.

Many other lifestyle factors are analyzed on the web pages of NormalBreathing.com.

8.13 Yoga is useful too (if you know how to breathe)

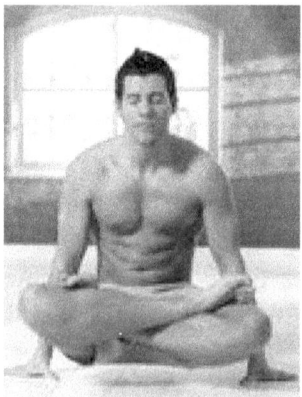

The answer to cystic fibrosis has been known even to yoga teachers for many centuries. The most comprehensive Sanskrit text on yoga "Shiva Sanhita" written several centuries ago states, "The truth-perceiving Yogi becomes free from disease, and sorrow or affliction; he never gets (putrid) perspiration, saliva and intestinal worms." Advanced Buteyko and yoga students can also testify that it is indeed so: with improved breath holding abilities, they naturally sleep less, have better digestion, no mucus production, and the smell of their perspiration changes from offensive to nearly neutral.

The presence of the faulty gene in CF does not in itself guarantee the development of CF symptoms and deteriorating health. It is the presence and development of chronic hyperventilation, tissue hypoxia and expression of the CFTR mutation gene that lead to classical symptoms of CF. Hence, the solution is to normalize the automatic breathing patterns and reverse negative effects due to hyperventilation.

9. Your program to defeat cystic fibrosis

9.1 Severe and moderate cystic fibrosis

For people with severe cystic fibrosis, up to 2 hours or more of daily breathing exercises with the Frolov breathing device or the Amazing DIY breathing device are required to start moving your CP up. If you decide to use Buteyko breathing exercises, you will need up to 3-4 hours for your daily breathwork.

People with only about 10-12 seconds current CP are often unable to do physical exercise and I suggest them to practice more breathing exercises so that to have around 15 seconds and then start walking with nose breathing only.

For example, a person with about 10 seconds CP can have serious problems due to shortness of breath or dyspnea during physical exercise (even walking). However, if this person spends 15 or 20 minutes with a breathing device, his or her CP will be about 15-17 seconds and walking or even power walking is much easier.

With about 20 seconds for the current CP, nearly all people with cystic fibrosis are able to do light jogging with strictly nasal breathing.

It is possible that some people get stuck with their CP growth. Even breathing exercises with devices do not produce significant CP changes (e.g., 3-5 s CP increase). This happens rarely and is most likely due to nutritional deficiencies (EFAs or fish oil, Ca, Mg and/or Zn) or too much inflammation and low production of cortisol. If you suspect cortisol deficiency, ask you doctor about the cortisol test. Buteyko doctors developed a special protocol how to find the optimum cortisol dose and how to safely wean off cortisol without any negative effects, but it is beyond the scope of this book to describe all these details.

Cystic Fibrosis

It is common and normal for people with cystic fibrosis to have slow or gradual CP progress. For example, someone with cystic fibrosis can gain only about 2-3 seconds per week for the morning CP progress. That means that your goal is to have at least 2-3 seconds for your average CP improvement after each week of breathing retraining. Be ready that the CP progress is often uneven and the morning CP numbers can fluctuate. It is important however that your average numbers steadily go up.

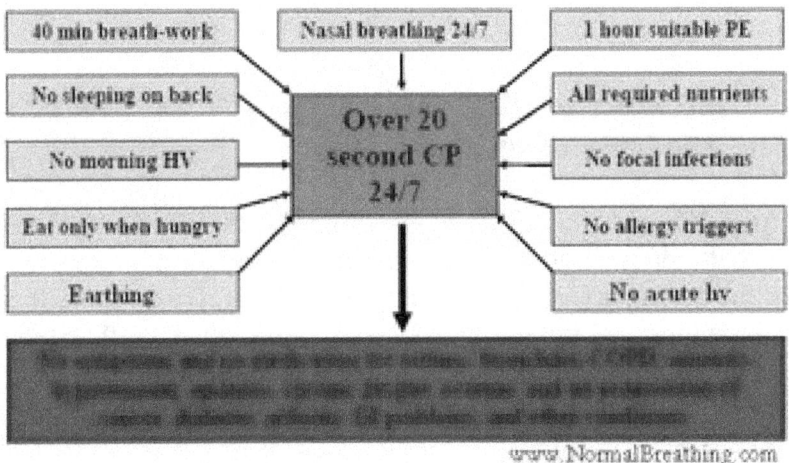

9.2 Mild cystic fibrosis

If the daily CP of the person is about 20 seconds (the morning test can be about 12-15 seconds) and the person is physically active, 1 hour per day with a breathing device (in total) should be enough to gradually increase your CP even to higher numbers. If you choose Buteyko breathing exercises, you may need up to 1.5-2 hours for your daily breathwork.

Your next goal is to get up to 30 seconds for the body oxygen test 24/7 and have nearly all symptoms of cystic fibrosis under control. There would be no production of new mucus, but be ready for intensive cleansing and discharges of old mucus (usually green or yellow, and can be with blood) from your sinuses and lungs.

When you get over 30 s for the morning CP, you will achieve partial restoration of the lungs and GI tract with either complete or almost complete elimination of chronic inflammation in various parts of the body.

Physical exercise becomes more and more important with higher CPs (and it is much easier and even pleasant to exercise at higher CPs), while there is no need to spend too much time for breathing exercises. Often, about 1 hour for Buteyko breathing exercises (which are easy to learn at higher CPs) are enough to move forward.

9.3 Your ultimate health goal is to have more than 50 s for the body oxygen test 24/7

For further progress, when you get about 32-35 seconds for the morning CP, you need to know the details of how to break through 40 s for the morning CP. I developed a fascinating program for this step in breathing retraining, and here are some changes that took place virtually in all people who get up to 50 s or more for their morning CP numbers.

Cystic Fibrosis

style factor:	Body oxygen < 30 s	Body oxygen > 50 s
ergy level	Medium, low, or very low	High
e to exercise	Not strong, but possible	Craving and joy of exercise
se with nose breathing	Hard or impossible	Easy and effortless
l mind states	Confusion, anxiety, depression	Focus, concentration, clarity
e, sugar and junk foods	Present	Absent
smoking, alcohol, and drugs	Possible	Absent
o eat raw foods	Weak and rare	Very common and natural
ect posture	Rare and requires efforts	Natural and automatic
Sleep	Often of poor quality; > 7 hours	Excellent quality; < 5 hours naturally

Dr. Artour Rakhimov

For more details about lifestyle modules, breathing exercises, sleep, physical exercise, digestive health, visit www.NormalBreathing.com

Success and easy breathing, Artour Rakhimov

Resources

www.NormalBreathing.com - the website with resources related to breathing exercise, modules with lifestyle changes, analysis of different breathing techniques, medical research related to chronic diseases, clinical trials, and other facts and details.

www.OxygenRemedy.org – probably the most comprehensive breathing retraining course that uses the most advanced breathing exercises and methods related to lifestyle changes

Amazing DIY Breathing Device (http://www.normalbreathing.com/book-DIY-breathing-device.php)– eBook (available PDF format or MOBI format for Kindle readers) with complete instructions how to make your own breathing device, practice breathing exercises, and make lifestyle changes for higher body oxygen test results.

www.youtube.com/artour2006 - Dr. Artour Rakhimov's YouTube Channel with about 40 videos (February 2012)

Bibliography

Bebök Z, Tousson A, Schwiebert LM, Venglarik CJ, Improved oxygenation promotes CFTR maturation and trafficking in MDCK monolayers, Am J Physiol Cell Physiol. 2001 Jan;280(1):C135-45.

Bell SC, Saunders MJ, Elborn JS, Shale DJ, Resting energy expenditure and oxygen cost of breathing in patients with cystic fibrosis, Thorax 1996 Feb; 51(2): 126-131.

Bonn JA, Readhead CP, Timmons BH, Enhanced adaptive behavioural response in agoraphobic patients pretreated with breathing retraining, Lancet 1984 Sep 22; 2(8404): 665-669.

Brihaye P, Jorissen M, Clement PA, Chronic rhinosinusitis in cystic fibrosis (mucoviscidosis), Acta Otorhinolaryngol Belg. 1997;51(4):323-37.

Brown EB, Physiological effects of hyperventilation 1953, Physiol Rev 33:445-471.

Browning IB, D'Alonzo GE, Tobin MJ, Importance of respiratory rate as an indicator of respiratory dysfunction in patients with cystic fibrosis, Chest. 1990 Jun;97(6):1317-21.

Buteyko KP, Dyomin DV, Odintsova MP, Ventilation of the Lungs and Arterial Vascular Tone Interconnection in Patients with High Blood Pressure and Angina Pectoris [In Ukrainian] Physiological Journal [Phyziologichny Zhurnal], 1965, vol. 11, N 5.

Buteyko KP, Odintsova MP, Nasonkina NS, Ventilation Test in Bronchial Asthma Patients [in Russian], Vrachebnoe Delo [Doctors Business], 1968, N4.

Carter AM, Grønlund J, Contribution of the Bohr effect to the fall in fetal PO2 caused by maternal alkalosis, J Perinat Med. 1985; 13(4): p.185-191.

Coetzee A, Holland D, Foëx P, Ryder A, Jones L, The effect of hypocapnia on coronary blood flow and myocardial function in the dog, Anesthesia and Analgesia 1984 Nov; 63(11): p. 991-997.

Dancey DR, Tullis ED, Heslegrave R, Thornley K, Hanly PJ, Sleep quality and daytime function in adults with cystic fibrosis and severe lung disease. Eur Respir J. 2002 Mar;19(3):504-10.

de Jong W, van Aalderen WM, Kraan J, Koëter GH, van der Schans CP, Inspiratory muscle training in patients with cystic fibrosis, Respir Med. 2001 Jan;95(1):31-6.

Delk KK, Gevirtz R, Hicks DA, Carden F, Rucker R, The effects of biofeedback assisted breathing retraining on lung functions in patients with cystic fibrosis, Chest. 1994 Jan;105(1):23-8.

diBella G, Scandariato G, Suriano O, Rizzo A, Oxygen affinity and Bohr effect responses to 2,3-diphosphoglycerate in equine and human blood, Res Vet Sci. 1996 May; 60(3): p. 272-275.

Divangahi M, Balghi H, Danialou G, Comtois AS, Demoule A, Ernest S, Haston C, Robert R, Hanrahan JW, Radzioch D, Petrof BJ, Lack of CFTR in skeletal muscle predisposes to muscle wasting and diaphragm muscle pump failure in cystic fibrosis mice, PLoS Genet. 2009 Jul; 5(7): e1000586.

Dodd JD, Barry SC, Barry RB, Gallagher CG, Skehan SJ, Masterson JB, Thin-section CT in patients with cystic fibrosis: correlation with peak exercise capacity and body mass index, Radiology. 2006 Jul;240(1):236-45.

Döring G, Worlitzsch D, Inflammation in cystic fibrosis and its management, Paediatr Respir Rev. 2000 Jun;1(2):101-6.

Dutton R, Levitzky M, Berkman R, Carbon dioxide and liver blood flow, Bull Eur Physiopathol Respir. 1976 Mar-Apr; 12(2): p. 265-273.

Dzhagarov BM, Kruk NN, The alkaline Bohr effect: regulation of O2 binding with triliganded hemoglobin Hb(O2)3 [Article in Russian] Biofizika. 1996 May-Jun; 41(3): p. 606-612.

Eby GA, Strong humming for one hour daily to terminate chronic rhinosinusitis in four days: a case report and hypothesis for action by stimulation of endogenous nasal nitric oxide production, Med Hypotheses. 2006;66(4):851-4. Epub 2006 Jan 10.

Enright S, Chatham K, Ionescu AA, Unnithan VB, Shale DJ, Inspiratory muscle training improves lung function and exercise capacity in adults with cystic fibrosis, Chest. 2004 Aug;126(2):405-11.

Esquivel E, Chaussain M, Plouin P, Ponsot G, Arthuis M, Physical exercise and voluntary hyperventilation in childhood absence epilepsy, Electroencephalogr Clin Neurophysiol 1991 Aug; 79(2): p. 127-132.

Fauroux B, Nicot F, Boelle PY, Boulé M, Clément A, Lofaso F, Bonora M, Mechanical limitation during CO2 rebreathing in young patients with cystic fibrosis, Respir Physiol Neurobiol. 2006 Oct 27;153(3):217-25. Epub 2005 Dec 27.

Fernald GW, Roberts MW, Boat TF, Cystic fibrosis: a current review, Pediatr Dent. 1990 Apr-May; 12(2):72-8.

Foëx P, Ryder WA, Effect of CO2 on the systemic and coronary circulations and on coronary sinus blood gas tensions, Bull Eur Physiopathol Respir 1979 Jul-Aug; 15(4): p.625-638.

Fortune JB, Feustel PJ, deLuna C, Graca L, Hasselbarth J, Kupinski AM, Cerebral blood flow and blood volume in response to O2 and CO2 changes in normal humans, J Trauma. 1995 Sep; 39(3): p. 463-471.

Frangolias DD, Wilcox PG, Predictability of oxygen desaturation during sleep in patients with cystic fibrosis : clinical, spirometric, and exercise parameters, Chest. 2001 Feb;119(2):434-41.

Fujita Y, Sakai T, Ohsumi A, Takaori M, Effects of hypocapnia and hypercapnia on splanchnic circulation and hepatic function in the beagle, Anesthesia and Analgesia 1989 Aug; 69(2): p. 152-157.

Genina VA, Hyperventilation in Bronchial Asthma Nosogenesis and its Treatment by Lung Ventilation Reduction [in Russian], Epidemiological Characteristics of Obstruction Lung Diseases in Various Professions. - Novosibirsk, 1982.

Gilmour DG, Douglas IH, Aitkenhead AR, Hothersall AP, Horton PW, Ledingham IM, Colon blood flow in the dog: effects of changes in arterial carbon dioxide tension, Cardiovasc Res 1980 Jan; 14(1): 11-20.

Gola G, Accinelli R, Morosi F, Orocraniofacial changes in young subjects with cystic fibrosis [Article in Italian], Mondo Ortod. 1989 Jan-Feb;14(1):11-7.

Gonzalez NC, Wood JG, Alveolar hypoxia-induced systemic inflammation: what low PO(2) does and does not do, Adv Exp Med Biol. 2010; 662: 27-32.

Grant BJ, Influence of Bohr-Haldane effect on steady-state gas exchange, J Appl Physiol. 1982 May; 52(5): p. 1330-1337.

Grasemann H, Knauer N, Büscher R, Hübner K, Drazen JM, Ratjen F, Airway nitric oxide levels in cystic fibrosis patients are related to a polymorphism in the neuronal nitric oxide synthase gene, Am J Respir Crit Care Med. 2000 Dec;162(6):2172-6.

Grasemann H, Ratjen F, Pulmonary metabolism of nitric oxide (NO) in patients with cystic fibrosis [Article in German], Pneumologie. 2002 Jun;56(6):376-81.

Guimbellot JS, Fortenberry JA, Siegal GP, Moore B, Wen H, Venglarik C, Chen YF, Oparil S, Sorscher EJ, Hong JS, Role of oxygen availability in CFTR expression and function, Am J Respir Cell Mol Biol. 2008 Nov;39(5):514-21.

Guzman JA, Kruse JA. Gut mucosal-arterial PCO2 gradient as an indicator of splanchnic perfusion during systemic hypo- and hypercapnia, Crit Care Med 1999; 27: p. 2760-2765.

Hart N, Tounian P, Clément A, Boulé M, Polkey MI, Lofaso F, Fauroux B, Nutritional status is an important predictor of diaphragm strength in young patients with cystic fibrosis, Am J Clin Nutr. 2004 Nov;80(5):1201-6.

Hatfield S, Belikoff B, Lukashev D, Sitkovsky M, Ohta A, The antihypoxia-adenosinergic pathogenesis as a result of collateral damage by overactive immune cells, J Leukoc Biol. 2009 Sep;86(3):545-8. Epub 2009 Jun 29.

Hellsing E, Brattström V, Strandvik B, Craniofacial morphology in children with cystic fibrosis, Eur J Orthod. 1992 Apr;14(2):147-51.

Holt PE, Andrews G, Provocation of panic: three elements of the panic reaction in four anxiety disorders, Behav Res Ther 1989; 27(3): p. 253-261.

Hughes RL, Mathie RT, Fitch W, Campbell D, Liver blood flow and oxygen consumption during hypocapnia and IPPV in the greyhound, J Appl Physiol. 1979 Aug; 47(2): p. 290-295.

Imtiyaz HZ, Simon MC, Hypoxia-inducible factors as essential regulators of inflammation, Curr Top Microbiol Immunol. 2010;345:105-20.

Jensen FB, Red blood cell pH, the Bohr effect, and other oxygenation-linked phenomena in blood O2 and CO2 transport, Acta Physiol Scand. 2004 Nov; 182(3): p. 215-227.

Karlsson T, Stjernström EL, Stjernström H, Norlén K, Wiklund L, Central and regional blood flow during hyperventilation. An experimental study in the pig, Acta Anaesthesiol Scand. 1994 Feb; 38(2): p.180-186.

Cystic Fibrosis

Keen C, Gustafsson P, Lindblad A, Wennergren G, Olin AC, Low levels of exhaled nitric oxide are associated with impaired lung function in cystic fibrosis, Pediatr Pulmonol. 2010 Mar;45(3):241-8.

Kennealy JA, McLennan JE, Loudon RG, McLaurin RL, Hyperventilation-induced cerebral hypoxia, Am Rev Respir Dis 1980, 122: p. 407-412.

Kister J, Marden MC, Bohn B, Poyart C, Functional properties of hemoglobin in human red cells: II. Determination of the Bohr effect, Respir Physiol. 1988 Sep; 73(3): p. 363-378.

Laffey JG & Kavanagh BP, Hypocapnia, New England Journal of Medicine 2002, 347(1) 43-53.

Lapennas GN, The magnitude of the Bohr coefficient: optimal for oxygen delivery, Respir Physiol. 1983 Nov; 54(2): p.161-172.

Liem KD, Kollée LA, Hopman JC, De Haan AF, Oeseburg B, The influence of arterial carbon dioxide on cerebral oxygenation and haemodynamics during ECMO in normoxaemic and hypoxaemic piglets, Acta Anaesthesiolica Scandanavica Supplement, 1995; 107: p.157-164.

Litchfield PM, A brief overview of the chemistry of respiration and the breathing heart wave, California Biofeedback, 2003 Spring, 19(1).

Lum LC, Hyperventilation: The Tip and the Iceberg, Journal of Psychosomatic Research, 1975, Vol. 19, pp. 375-383.

Lum LC, Hyperventilation and Anxiety State, Journal of the Royal Society of Medicine, 1981 (74) 1-4.

Liem KD, Kollée LA, Hopman JC, De Haan AF, Oeseburg B, The influence of arterial carbon dioxide on cerebral oxygenation and haemodynamics during ECMO in normoxaemic and hypoxaemic piglets, Acta Anaesthesiol Scand Suppl. 1995; 107: p.157-164.

Macey PM, Woo MA, Harper RM, Hyperoxic brain effects are normalized by addition of CO2, PLoS Medicine, 2007 May; 4(5): p. e173.

McKone EF, Barry SC, Fitzgerald MX, Gallagher CG, Role of arterial hypoxemia and pulmonary mechanics in exercise limitation in adults with cystic fibrosis, J Appl Physiol. 2005 Sep;99(3):1012-8. Epub 2005 Apr 28.

Mojsoski N, Pavicic F, Study of bronchial reactivity using dry, cold air and eucapnic hyperventilation [in Serbo-Croatian], Plucne Bolesti 1990 Jan-Jun; 42(1-2): p. 38-42.

Nakao K, Ohgushi M, Yoshimura M, Morooka K, Okumura K, Ogawa H, Kugiyama K, Oike Y, Fujimoto K, Yasue H, Hyperventilation as a specific test for diagnosis of coronary artery spasm. Am J Cardiol 1997 Sep 1; 80(5): p. 545-549.

Nardi AE, Valenca AM, Nascimento I, Mezzasalma MA, Lopes FL, Zin WA, Hyperventilation in panic disorder patients and healthy first-degree relatives, Braz J Med Biol Res 2000 Nov; 33(11): p. 1317-1323.

Nunn JF. Applied respiratory physiology, 1987, 3rd ed. London: Butterworths.

Okazaki K, Okutsu Y, Fukunaga A, Effect of carbon dioxide (hypocapnia and hypercapnia) on tissue blood flow and oxygenation of liver, kidneys and skeletal muscle in the dog, Masui 1989 Apr, 38 (4): p. 457-464.

Okazaki K, Hashimoto K, Okutsu Y, Okumura F, Effect of arterial carbon dioxide tension on regional myocardial tissue oxygen tension in the dog [Article in Japanese], Masui 1991 Nov; 40(11): p. 1620-1624.

Okazaki K, Hashimoto K, Okutsu Y, Okumura F, Effect of carbon dioxide (hypocapnia and hypercapnia) on regional myocardial tissue oxygen tension in dogs with coronary stenosis [Article in Japanese],

Masui 1992 Feb; 41(2): p. 221-224.

Pinet C, Cassart M, Scillia P, et al. Function and bulk of respiratory and limb muscles in patients with cystic fibrosis. Am J Respir Crit Care Med 2003; 168: 989–994.

Primiano FP Jr, Saidel GM, Montague FW Jr, Kruse KL, Green CG, Horowitz JG, Water vapour and temperature dynamics in the upper airways of normal and CF subjects, Eur Respir J. 1988 May;1(5):407-14.

Ranganathan SC, Goetz I, Hoo AF, Lum S, Castle R, Stocks J, Assessment of tidal breathing parameters in infants with cystic fibrosis, Eur Respir J. 2003 Nov;22(5):761-6.

Rolla G, Heffler E, Bommarito L, Bergia R, Ferrero N, Exhaled nitric oxide as a marker of diseases [Article in Italian], Recenti Prog Med. 2005 Dec;96(12):634-40.

Ryan S, Taylor CT, McNicholas WT, Systemic inflammation: a key factor in the pathogenesis of cardiovascular complications in obstructive sleep apnoea syndrome? Thorax. 2009 Jul; 64(7): 631-636.

Safronova O, Morita I, Transcriptome remodeling in hypoxic inflammation, J Dent Res. 2010 May; 89(5):430-44.

Salvatore D, D'Andria M, Effects of salmeterol on arterial oxyhemoglobin saturations in patients with cystic fibrosis, Pediatr Pulmonol. 2002 Jul;34(1):11-5.

Santiago TV & Edelman NH, Brain blood flow and control of breathing, in Handbook of Physiology, Section 3: The respiratory system, vol. II, ed. by AP Fishman. American Physiological Society, Betheda, Maryland, 1986, p. 163-179.

Scadding G, Nitric oxide in the airways, Curr Opin Otolaryngol Head Neck Surg. 2007 Aug;15(4):258-63.

Sitkovsky MV, T regulatory cells: hypoxia-adenosinergic suppression and re-direction of the immune response, Trends Immunol. 2009 Mar;30(3):102-8. Epub 2009 Feb 7.

Skippen P, Seear M, Poskitt K, et al. Effect of hyperventilation on regional cerebral blood flow in head-injured children. Crit Care Med 1997, 25: p. 1402-1409.

Sumbayev VV, Nicholas SA, Hypoxia-inducible factor 1 as one of the "signaling drivers" of Toll-like receptor-dependent and allergic inflammation, Arch Immunol Ther Exp (Warsz). 2010 Aug;58(4):287-94. Epub 2010 May 26.

Szeinberg A, England S, Mindorff C, Fraser IA, Levison H, Maximal inspiratory and expiratory pressures are reduced in hyperinflated, malnpourished, young adult male patients with cystic fibrosis. Am Rev Respir Dis 1985; 132: 766–769.

Tepper RS, Skatrud B, Dempsey JA, Ventilation and oxygenation changes during sleep in cystic fibrosis, Chest 1983; 84; p. 388-393.

Törnberg DC, Marteus H, Schedin U, Alving K, Lundberg JO, Weitzberg E, Nasal and oral contribution to inhaled and exhaled nitric oxide: a study in tracheotomized patients, Eur Respir J. 2002 May;19(5):859-64.

Tsuda Y, Kimura K, Yoneda S, Hartmann A, Etani H, Hashikawa K, Kamada T, Effect of hypocapnia on cerebral oxygen metabolism and blood flow in ischemic cerebrovascular disorders, Eur Neurol. 1987; 27(3): p.155-163.

Tyuma I, The Bohr effect and the Haldane effect in human hemoglobin, Jpn J Physiol. 1984; 34(2): p.205-216.

Villa MP, Pagani J, Lucidi V, Palamides S, Ronchetti R, Nocturnal oximetry in infants with cystic fibrosis, Arch Dis Child. 2001 Jan;84(1):50-54.

Ward SA, Tomezsko JL, Holsclaw DS, Paolone AM, Energy

expenditure and substrate utilization in adults with cystic fibrosis and diabetes mellitus, Am J Clin Nutr. 1999 May;69(5):913-9.

Weitzberg E, Lundberg JO, Humming greatly increases nasal nitric oxide, Am J Respir Crit Care Med. 2002 Jul 15;166(2):144-5.

Wexels JC, Myhre ES, Mjøs OD, Effects of carbon dioxide and pH on myocardial blood-flow and metabolism in the dog, Clin Physiol. 1985 Dec; 5(6): p.575-588.

Wheatley CM, Foxx-Lupo WT, Cassuto NA, Wong EC, Daines CL, Morgan WJ, Snyder EM, Impaired lung diffusing capacity for nitric oxide and alveolar-capillary membrane conductance results in oxygen desaturation during exercise in patients with cystic fibrosis, J Cyst Fibros. 2011 Jan;10(1):45-53. Epub 2010 Nov 2.

Wirrel CW, Camfield PR, Gordon KE, Camfield CS, Dooley JM, and Hanna BD, Will a critical level of hypocapnia always induce an absence seizure? Epilepsia 1996; 37(5): p. 459-462.

Young AC, Wilson JW, Kotsimbos TC, Naughton MT, The impact of nocturnal oxygen desaturation on quality of life in cystic fibrosis, J Cyst Fibros. 2011 Mar;10(2):100-6.

Zheng W, Kuhlicke J, Jäckel K, Eltzschig HK, Singh A, Sjöblom M, Riederer B, Weinhold C, Seidler U, Colgan SP, Karhausen J, Hypoxia inducible factor-1 (HIF-1)-mediated repression of cystic fibrosis transmembrane conductance regulator (CFTR) in the intestinal epithelium, FASEB J. 2009 Jan;23(1):204-13.

Dr. Artour Rakhimov

About the author: Dr. Artour Rakhimov

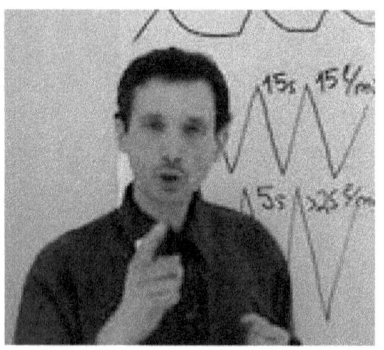

 * High School Honor student (Grade "A" for all exams)
 * Moscow University Honor student (Grade "A" for all exams)
 * Moscow University PhD (Math/Physics), accepted in Canada and the UK
 * Winner of many regional competitions in mathematics, chess and sport orienteering (during teenage and University years)
 * Good classical piano-player: Chopin, Bach, Tchaikovsky, Beethoven, Strauss (up to now)
 * Former captain of the ski-O varsity team and member of the cross-country skiing varsity team of the Moscow State University, best student teams of the USSR
 * Former individual coach of world-elite athletes from Soviet (Russian) and Finnish national teams who took gold and silver medals during World Championships
 * Total distance covered by running, cross country skiing, and swimming: over 100,000 km or over 2.5 loops around the Earth
 * Joined Religious Society of Friends (Quakers) in 2001
 * Author of the publication which won Russian National 1998 Contest of scientific and methodological sport papers
 * Author of the books, as well as an author of the bestselling Amazon books:
 - *"Oxygenate Yourself: Breathe Less" (Buteyko Books; 94 pages; ISBN: 0954599683; 2008; Hardcover)*
 - *"Cystic Fibrosis Reversed" 2012 - Amazon Kindle book*
 - *"Doctors Who Cure Cancer" 2012 - Amazon Kindle book*

Cystic Fibrosis

- "Yoga Benefits Are in Breathing Less" 2012 - Amazon Kindle book
- "Crohn's Disease and Colitis: Hidden Triggers and Symptoms" 2012 - Amazon Kindle book
- "How to Use Frolov Breathing Device (Instructions)" - 2012 - PDF and Amazon book (120 pages)
- "Amazing DIY Breathing Device" - 2010-2012 - PDF and Amazon book
- "What Science and Professor Buteyko Teach Us About Breathing" 2002
- "Breathing, Health and Quality of Life" 2004 (91 pages; Translated in Danish and Finnish)
- "Doctor Buteyko Lecture at the Moscow State University" 2009 (55 pages; Translation from Russian with Dr. A. Rakhimov's comments)
- "Normal Breathing: the Key to Vital Health" 2009 (The most comprehensive world's book on Buteyko breathing retraining method; over 190,000 words; 305 pages)

* Author of the world's largest website devoted to breathing, breathing techniques, and breathing retraining (www.NormalBreathing.com)
* Author of numerous YouTube videos (http://www.youtube.com/user/artour2006)
* Buteyko breathing teacher (since 2002 up to now) and trainer
* Inventor of the Amazing DIY breathing device and numerous contributions to breathing retraining
* Whistleblower and investigator of mysterious murder-suicides, massacres and other crimes organized worldwide by GULAG KGB agents using the fast total mind control method
* Practitioner of the New Decision Therapy and Kantillation
* Level 2 Trainer of the New Decision Therapy
* Health writer and health educator